THE COMPLETE HIGH-PROTEIN HIGH-FIBER MEAL PREP GUIDE

Wholesome, Tasty Meals and 4 Step-By-Step Meal Prepping Guides for Boosting Vitality | Full Color Edition

Betty J. Lawson

Manufactured in the United States of America
Interior and Cover Designer: Danielle Rees
Art Producer: Brooke White
Editor: Aaliyah Lyons
Production Editor: Sienna Adams
Production Manager: Sarah Johnson
Photography: Michael Smith

TABLE OF CONTENTS

TABLE OF CONTENTS

INTRODUCTION

I've got to be honest—my journey into meal prepping didn't start with some grand health awakening. Nope. It began when I realized how much time (and money) I was wasting on takeout and snacks. I'd be rushing around, juggling work, social life, and everything in between, and somehow, my meals always ended up being a second thought. Sound familiar?

One day, after what felt like my hundredth overpriced salad that left me hungry an hour later, I decided enough was enough. I needed food that actually kept me full, gave me energy, and didn't make me want to nap at 3 p.m. That's when I dove into the world of high-protein, high-fiber meals. At first, I was clueless. I thought eating healthy meant bland chicken and steamed broccoli—every single day. But as I started experimenting in the kitchen, I realized that healthy meals could be tasty, satisfying, and yes, even easy to prep ahead.

I started with a few simple recipes, and let me tell you, there's something so rewarding about opening the fridge and seeing all your meals ready to go. No more last-minute "what's for dinner?" panic! My energy levels shot up, and I didn't feel like I was starving between meals anymore. Plus, my grocery bills? Way more manageable.

Now, I'm not some culinary wizard, but I've learned a few tricks that work wonders, and I'm here to share them with you.

My goal with this guide is simple: to help you find the balance between delicious, nutritious, and practical. So, whether you're new to meal prep or looking to spice things up, I've got you covered. Let's make healthy eating something you actually look forward to!

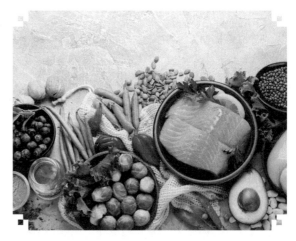

DEDICATION

I want to give a huge shoutout to my amazing BFF, Ava! When I first mentioned I wanted to start meal prepping, I had no idea where to begin. Little did I know, Ava had been rocking the healthy eating game for years! She generously shared her tips, recipes, and experiences with me, making my journey to eating healthier so much easier. Thanks to her, I've been able to dive right in and make healthy eating a part of my routine. Ava, you're truly the best, and I'm so grateful to have you by my side on this journey!

CHAPTER 1: THE EASY WAY TO HIGH-PROTEIN, HIGH-FIBER EATING

THE POWER OF HIGH-PROTEIN, HIGH-FIBER MEALS

If you're looking to fuel your body right, there's no better combo than protein and fiber. Together, they create a powerhouse of benefits that can keep you feeling energized, full, and healthy. Let's break down why protein and fiber matter and how they work together to transform your diet.

✓ WHY PROTEIN MATTERS: ENERGY, STRENGTH, AND SATIETY

Protein is often called the building block of life, and for a good reason. It's crucial for repairing tissues, building muscle, and producing essential hormones and enzymes. But beyond its biological roles, protein has some pretty cool benefits when it comes to how you feel daily. Ever notice how a high-carb breakfast leaves you starving by mid-morning, while a protein-rich meal keeps you going until lunch? That's because protein takes longer to digest, providing a steady energy release rather than a quick spike and crash.

Eating enough protein is key for maintaining and building muscle, especially if you're active. Whether you're hitting the gym or just trying to stay strong and fit, protein helps repair muscle fibers that break down during exercise, supporting recovery and growth. And let's not forget satiety—protein is fantastic at making you feel full. It sends signals to your brain that say, "Hey, I'm good," which can help control hunger and reduce mindless snacking.

✓ THE ROLE OF FIBER: DIGESTION, WEIGHT MANAGEMENT, AND GUT HEALTH

Fiber might not sound as exciting as protein, but it's just as important. There are two types of fiber—soluble and insoluble—and both play unique roles in keeping your body in top shape. Soluble fiber dissolves in water to form a gel-like substance that can help lower cholesterol and regulate blood sugar levels. On the other hand, insoluble fiber doesn't dissolve; instead, it adds bulk to your stool, helping keep things moving through your digestive system and preventing constipation.

But fiber's benefits go beyond digestion. A high-fiber diet can help with weight management because fiber adds bulk to your meals without adding extra calories. This means you can eat satisfying portions and feel full longer, which can naturally help reduce overall calorie intake. Plus, fiber is a superstar for gut health. It acts like a prebiotic, feeding the good bacteria in your gut. A healthy gut microbiome is linked to everything from better digestion to improved mood and immune function.

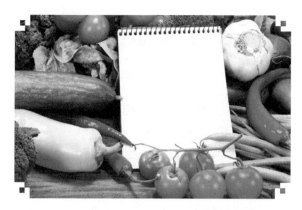 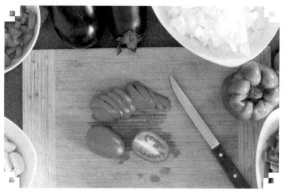

✓ HOW COMBINING PROTEIN AND FIBER CAN TRANSFORM YOUR DIET

Now, here's where the magic happens—combining protein and fiber in your meals. When you pair these two nutrients, you're setting yourself up for a steady stream of energy, balanced blood sugar levels, and sustained fullness. Imagine starting your day with a breakfast that's both high in protein and fiber, like Greek yogurt with berries and a sprinkle of chia seeds. You get the muscle-supporting benefits of protein and the digestive support of fiber in one delicious bowl.

The synergy between protein and fiber also helps keep cravings at bay. When your meals are balanced with both nutrients, you're less likely to experience the highs and lows of blood sugar spikes, which often lead to sugar cravings and overeating. Instead, you feel satisfied, energized, and ready to take on the day without constantly thinking about your next meal.

And it's not just about weight management or muscle building—this combination can support overall health. A diet rich in protein and fiber has been linked to better heart health, reduced inflammation, and improved cholesterol levels. So, it's more than just a diet; it's a lifestyle that supports long-term wellness.

MEAL PREP SUCCESS: TIPS AND TRICKS

Getting into meal prep might seem like a big task at first, but trust me, once you get the hang of it, you'll wonder how you ever managed without it. It's all about setting yourself up for success with the right tools, understanding the different approaches to prepping, and knowing how to store your meals to keep them fresh and tasty. Here's how to master meal prep like a pro!

▸ BASIC TOOLS AND ESSENTIALS YOU'LL NEED

First things first, let's talk about the gear. You don't need a kitchen full of fancy gadgets to start meal prepping, but having a few basics will make your life a lot easier. Here's a quick rundown of what you'll need:

Quality Containers

Invest in a set of durable, reusable containers. Look for ones that are BPA-free, microwave-safe, and leak-proof. A mix of sizes will help you store everything from individual snacks to full meals. Glass containers are great for reheating and don't stain like plastic.

Measuring Cups and Spoons

These are a must for portion control. Whether you're counting calories or just trying to make sure your meals are balanced, having accurate measurements helps you stay on track.

A Sharp Chef's Knife and Cutting Board

Meal prep involves a lot of chopping, slicing, and dicing, so a good knife and a sturdy cutting board are essential. A sharp knife not only makes prep faster but also safer.

Non-Stick Sheet Pans and Baking Trays

Roasting is a meal prepper's best friend. Sheet pans are perfect for cooking large batches of veggies, proteins, or even entire sheet pan dinners.

A Slow Cooker or Instant Pot

These gadgets can save you time and effort. They're perfect for preparing large batches of soups, stews, or shredded chicken with minimal hands-on time.

Labels and a Marker

Keeping track of what you've prepped and when is key to avoiding food waste. Label your containers with the contents and the date to know what to eat first.

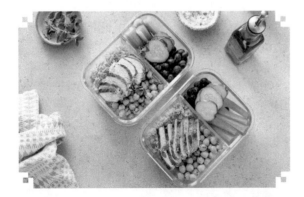

▶ STORAGE SOLUTIONS FOR MAXIMUM FRESHNESS

Keeping your prepped meals fresh is crucial, not only for taste but also for safety. Here are some storage tips to make sure your meals stay at their best:

- **Cool Quickly:** After cooking, let your food cool down a bit before sealing it in containers. This helps prevent condensation, which can lead to soggy food and bacterial growth. However, don't leave food out for too long—two hours is the maximum.

- **Use Airtight Containers:** Air is the enemy of freshness. Airtight containers help prevent oxidation and keep food from drying out. If you're storing soups or sauces, consider leaving a little space at the top of the container for expansion if you're planning to freeze them.

- **Master the Freezer Game:** The freezer is your best friend for long-term storage. Portion out meals into freezer-safe containers or bags, label them with the contents and date, and stack them neatly. Foods like cooked grains, soups, and proteins freeze well and can be reheated easily.

- **Store with Purpose:** Keep foods that spoil faster—like salads or cut fruits—toward the front of the fridge, where they're easy to grab and eat first. Hardier items like cooked grains, beans, or roasted veggies can be stored in the back or even in the freezer.

- **Plan for Rotation:** Follow the "first in, first out" rule. Use the oldest items first to avoid waste and keep your meals tasting fresh.

THE ULTIMATE FOOD LIST

When it comes to a high-protein, high-fiber diet, knowing which foods to focus on is key to success. The right mix of proteins, fiber-rich foods, and healthy fats will not only fuel your body but also keep you satisfied and energized. Here's a breakdown of the best foods to include in your meal prep routine.

Proteins That Pack a Punch

Protein is essential for muscle repair, energy, and keeping you full. Here's a look at some of the best protein sources you can add to your diet:

Lean Meats and Poultry

Think chicken breast, turkey, lean cuts of beef, and pork tenderloin. These options are low in fat but high in protein, making them perfect for building muscle and keeping hunger at bay. Grilling, baking, or stir-frying are great ways to prepare these meats without adding extra fat.

Plant-Based Proteins: Beans, Lentils, and Tofu

For those who prefer plant-based options, beans, lentils, and tofu are excellent choices. Not only are they rich in protein, but they

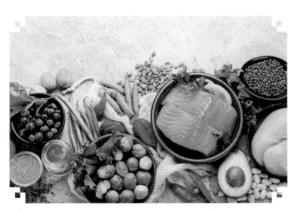

also come with a hefty dose of fiber, making them a two-in-one nutritional powerhouse. Lentils are great in soups and salads, beans can be added to chili or burritos, and tofu is perfect for stir-fries and curries.

Seafood and Fish: Rich in Protein and Omega-3s

Salmon, tuna, mackerel, and sardines aren't just high in protein—they're also packed with omega-3 fatty acids, which support heart health and reduce inflammation. Fish cooks quickly and can be baked, grilled, or poached for an easy, nutritious meal.

Dairy and Alternatives: Greek Yogurt, Cottage Cheese, and More

Dairy products like Greek yogurt, cottage cheese, and cheese are convenient, protein-rich snacks or additions to meals. They provide a good amount of calcium, too. If you're lactose intolerant or prefer non-dairy options, look for fortified plant-based alternatives like almond, soy, or coconut yogurt.

Fiber-Rich Essentials

Fiber is your secret weapon for digestion, weight management, and overall health. Here's where to find it:

Whole Grains: Quinoa, Brown Rice, Oats, and Beyond

Whole grains like quinoa, brown rice, oats, bulgur, and barley are fantastic sources of fiber. They are versatile and can be the base for a wide variety of dishes, from breakfast bowls to dinner plates. Whole grains not only help keep you full but also provide sustained energy throughout the day.

Vegetables High in Fiber: Broccoli, Spinach, Brussels Sprouts, etc.

Vegetables like broccoli, spinach, Brussels sprouts, carrots, and kale are packed with fiber and essential nutrients like vitamins A, C, and K. Roasting, steaming, or sautéing them can help retain their nutrients and add flavor. Don't be shy about piling these onto your plate—your body will thank you!

Fruits That Fuel: Berries, Apples, Pears, and More

Berries (like blueberries, raspberries, and strawberries), apples, pears, and oranges are high in fiber, antioxidants, and vitamins. They're perfect for snacking or adding to smoothies, salads, and yogurt. These fruits help keep you hydrated and offer natural sweetness without added sugars.

Nuts and Seeds: Chia, Flaxseeds, Almonds, and Walnuts

Nuts and seeds are not only good sources of protein but are also loaded with fiber and healthy fats. Chia seeds and flaxseeds can be added to smoothies, oatmeal, or baked goods for an extra fiber boost. Almonds, walnuts, and pistachios make for great snacks or crunchy toppings on salads and yogurt.

Healthy Fats for Flavor and Satiety

Healthy fats are crucial for maintaining cell structure, supporting brain health, and adding flavor to your meals. They also help you stay full longer.

- **Avocado, Olive Oil, and Nuts:** Avocado is a creamy, delicious way to add healthy fats to your diet. It's great in salads, on toast, or as a topping for proteins. Olive oil is another must-have; it's ideal for salad dressings, sautéing, or roasting vegetables. A handful of nuts like almonds, cashews, or walnuts can provide a quick dose of healthy fats and a satisfying crunch.

- **Incorporating Seeds for Added Benefits:** Seeds like chia, flaxseeds, sunflower seeds, and pumpkin seeds are small but mighty. They're packed with omega-3 fatty acids, protein, and fiber. Sprinkle them on your salads, blend them into smoothies, or add them to homemade granola for an extra nutritional kick.

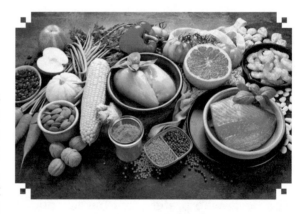

Incorporating high-protein, high-fiber foods into your diet is a game-changer for both health and convenience. By focusing on these nutrient-packed options, you can fuel your body efficiently, manage hunger, and support overall well-being. Embrace these essentials, and you'll find meal prep becomes a seamless part of your routine.

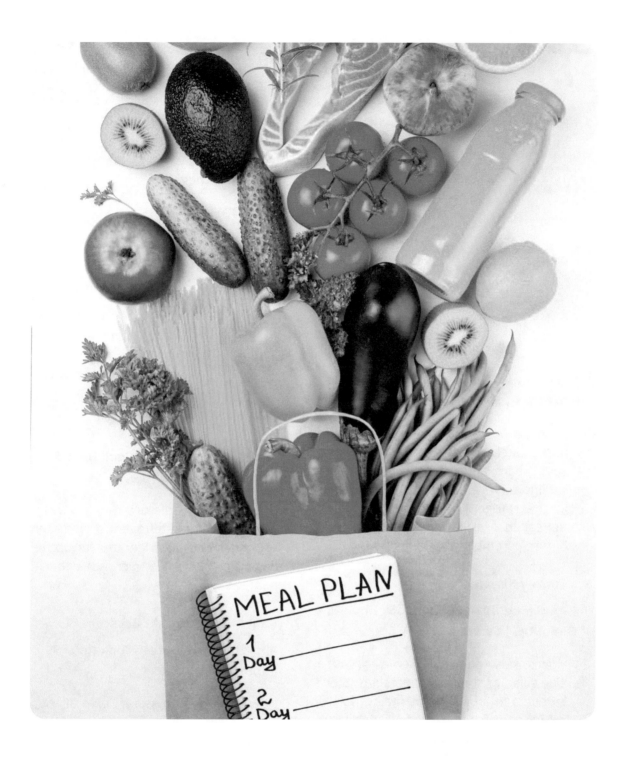

CHAPTER 2: 4-WEEK MEAL PLAN

MEAL PLAN WEEK 1

1. Peanut Butter And Banana Mug Muffins

Prep time: 5 minutes | Cook time: 5 minutes | Serves 3

How to serve and store: Serve warm straight from the mugs or turned out onto a plate. Store muffins individually in airtight containers in the refrigerator for up to 3 days. Reheat in the microwave for 20-30 seconds before serving.

2. Breakfast Tostadas

Prep time: 10 minutes | Cook time: 20 minutes | Serves 4

How to serve and store: Serve immediately, topped with fresh salsa, sour cream, and cilantro. Store leftover cauliflower rice in an airtight container in the refrigerator for up to 3 days. Reheat in a skillet over medium heat before assembling tostadas.

3. Turkey Rissoles

Prep time: 10 minutes | Cook time: 25 minutes | Serves 4

How to serve and store: Serve hot with a side salad or steamed vegetables. Store leftovers in an airtight container in the refrigerator for up to 4 days. Reheat in the oven at 350°F for 10-15 minutes or until warmed through.

4. Beef And Broccoli Roast

Prep time: 10 minutes | Cook time: 4 hours 30 minutes | Serves 2

How to serve and store: Serve hot over rice or noodles. Store leftovers in an airtight container in the refrigerator for up to 3 days. Reheat in the microwave or in a skillet over medium heat until warmed through.

5. Asian Seafood Stir-Fry

Prep time: 10 minutes | Cook time:15 minutes |Serves 4

How to serve and store: Serve immediately with rice or noodles. Store leftovers in an airtight container in the refrigerator for up to 2 days. Reheat in a wok or skillet over medium heat until hot.

6. Cilantro Lime Rice

Prep time: 5 minutes |Cook time: 5 minutes| Serves 4

How to serve and store: Serve warm as a side dish. Store leftovers in an airtight container in the refrigerator for up to 3 days. Reheat in the microwave for 1-2 minutes before serving.

7. Café Mocha Protein Bars

Prep time: 5 minutes |Cook time: 35 minutes| Serves 4

How to serve and store: Serve at room temperature. Store bars in an airtight container at room temperature for up to 3 days or refrigerate for up to 1 week. Enjoy chilled or at room temperature.

8. Lemon-Poppyseed Cookies

Prep time: 5 minutes | Cook time: 15 minutes | Serves 4

How to serve and store: Serve at room temperature, plain or with a glass of unsweetened, plant-based milk. Store cookies in an airtight container at room temperature for up to 5 days.

WEEK 1 SHOPPING LIST

Pantry:

- Nonstick cooking spray
- Coconut oil (1 tablespoon)
- Olive oil (2 tablespoons)
- Ground cinnamon (1½ teaspoons)
- Ground paprika (2 teaspoons)
- Ground coriander (1 teaspoon)
- Ground oregano (2 teaspoons)
- Ground cumin (1 teaspoon)
- Pink Himalayan salt (to taste)
- Kosher salt (to taste)
- Freshly ground black pepper (to taste)
- Soy sauce or coconut aminos (¼ cup + 1 tablespoon)
- Toasted sesame oil (1 teaspoon + 4 teaspoons)
- Coconut aminos (1 tablespoon)
- Rice wine (2 tablespoons)
- Baking powder (¼ teaspoon)
- Cocoa powder (1 teaspoon)
- Ground coffee (1 tablespoon)
- Stevia (1 packet)
- Monk fruit sweetener (¾ cup)

Grain:

- Quick oats (¾ cup)
- Oat bran (¼ cup)
- Dry oatmeal (¾ cup)

Fruit:

- Ripe banana (1)

- Avocados (2)
- Lime, juiced and zested (1 medium)
- Lemon juice (from 1 lemon)

Dairy:

- Egg whites (¾ cup + 6 large)
- Sour cream (1 cup)

Vegetables, Herbs, and Spices:

- Jicama (1, peeled)
- Cauliflower rice (4 cups + 10 ounces)
- Fresh salsa (1 cup, divided)
- Fresh cilantro, chopped (¼ cup + ½ cup)
- Scallion, chopped (1)
- Yellow onion, sliced (½ cup)
- Asparagus spears, sliced (1 cup)
- Celery, chopped (½ cup)
- Enoki mushrooms (½ cup)
- Fresh parsley, chopped (1 tablespoon)
- Fresh grated lemon zest (3 tablespoons)

Nuts and Seeds:

- Chia seeds (4 tablespoons)
- Poppy seeds (1 tablespoon)
- Dry roasted peanuts, chopped (½ cup)
- Almond butter (1 cup)

Protein:

- Ground turkey (1 pound)
- Beef chuck roast (1 pound)
- Bay scallops (1 pound)
- Chocolate protein powder (1 scoop)
- Peanut butter (3 tablespoons)

WEEK 1 MEAL PREPARATION

To make Peanut Butter and Banana Mug Muffins, first spray 3 large mugs with nonstick cooking spray to prevent the muffins from sticking. Mix the banana, egg whites, oats, peanut butter, vanilla, and cinnamon in a medium bowl. Then, fold in the chocolate chips if you choose to use them. Next, divide the batter equally among the 3 mugs and microwave each mug on high for 2 minutes. Ensure that the muffins are cooked through and the top is firm to the touch before removing them from the microwave. Use a butter knife to free the sides of the muffins from the mugs, and then turn the mugs upside down to shake the muffins onto a plate. Let the muffins cool. Finally, place each muffin into a separate airtight storage container and seal them to keep the muffins fresh.

Prepare for Breakfast Tostadas while the Muffins are cooking. Start by slicing the jicama into thin discs using a mandoline or a sharp chef's knife and set them aside. Next, warm some coconut oil in a large skillet over medium heat. Then, add the cauliflower rice, paprika, coriander, oregano, and cumin to the skillet. Cook the mixture, stirring frequently and allowing any excess water to evaporate, for approximately 12 minutes. Once the cauliflower becomes tender, remove the skillet from the heat. To assemble the tostadas, arrange the jicama slices on a serving platter. Top each slice with a generous spoonful of cooked cauliflower, some slices of creamy avocado, a dollop of fresh salsa, a swirl of sour cream, and a sprinkle of fresh cilantro.

While the tostadas are cooking, prepare for Turkey Rissoles. Start by preheating the oven to 350°F and lining a baking sheet with aluminum foil. In a medium-sized bowl, combine the ground turkey, finely chopped scallions, minced garlic, salt, and pepper until the ingredients are well mixed. Form the mixture into 8 evenly sized patties and gently flatten them. Next, place ground almonds in a shallow bowl and coat each turkey patty with the almonds. Heat olive oil in a large skillet over medium heat and carefully brown the patties on both sides for approximately 10 minutes. Once browned, transfer the patties to the prepared baking sheet and bake them in the oven until they are fully cooked, remembering to flip them over once during the process. This should take about 15 minutes in total.

Prepare for Beef And Broccoli Roast while the turkey is cooking. Before you start, make sure the crock insert is in place in the slow cooker, and preheat it by setting it to low. Begin by laying out a cutting board and seasoning the chuck roast generously with pink Himalayan salt and black pepper. Then, place the roast in thin pieces in the slow cooker. Next, in a small bowl, combine the beef broth, soy sauce, and sesame oil. Once mixed, pour the mixture over the beef in the slow cooker to infuse the meat with flavor. Cover the slow cooker and let the beef cook on low for 4 hours. After this time, add the frozen broccoli to the slow cooker and continue cooking for 30 minutes. Add beef broth to maintain the desired consistency if the dish needs more liquid. Once the cooking is complete, serve the dish hot.

While the beef and broccoli roast is inside the slow cooker, prepare for Asian Seafood Stir-Fry. Begin by heating 1 teaspoon of sesame oil in a wok over a medium-high flame. Sauté the onion until it reaches a perfect balance of crisp-tenderness and translucency, and then set it aside. Next, add another teaspoon of sesame oil to the wok and sauté the asparagus and celery until they are crisp-tender, creating a delightful contrast of textures; reserve them as well. Then, using another teaspoon of sesame oil, cook the mushrooms for 2 minutes until they soften, and set them aside. Finally, heat the remaining teaspoon of sesame oil and cook the bay scallops until they turn a beautiful opaque color. Combine all the reserved vegetables back into the wok and add the remaining ingredients, giving everything a good toss to ensure it's well-mixed.

Prepare for Cilantro Lime Rice while the Asian seafood is cooking. Combine the riced cauliflower with water in a generously sized microwave-safe bowl and microwave it for 3 to 5 minutes or until the cauliflower reaches the desired level of softness. Once done, take it out and incorporate the lime juice, zest, and cilantro into the bowl, making sure to mix everything thoroughly before serving.

While cooking cilantro lime rice, prepare for Café Mocha Protein Bars. Start by preheating your oven to 350°F. Then, grab your blender and combine all the ingredients until you have a smooth mixture. Next, take a greased 10" × 13" baking dish and transfer the mixture into it. Pop the dish into the preheated oven and bake for about 30 minutes. Once done, allow the bars to cool before cutting them into 4 equal pieces.

Prepare for Lemon-Poppyseed Cookies while the mocha protein bars are inside the oven. start by preheating the oven to 350°F and greasing a baking sheet with cooking spray. In a large mixing bowl, combine the rich almond butter with the natural sweetness of monk fruit sweetener, wholesome chia seeds, fragrant lemon zest, refreshing lemon juice, and crunchy poppy seeds. Mix everything well, using your hands to knead the mixture thoroughly. Next, roll pieces of the dough into cookie-size balls and place them on the prepared baking sheet, making sure to space them evenly to allow for spreading during baking. Bake the cookies for approximately 8 minutes or until they turn golden. Once baked to perfection, transfer the cookies to a cooling rack. These delicious cookies can be enjoyed as they are or paired with your favorite unsweetened, plant-based milk for a delightful treat.

MEAL PLAN WEEK 2

1. **Pancake "Cake"**

   Prep time: 5 minutes | Cook time: 20 minutes | Serves 4

   How to serve and store: Serve warm, topped with additional butter if desired. Store leftovers in an airtight container in the refrigerator for up to 3 days. Reheat in the microwave for 20-30 seconds before serving.

2. **Kale-Avocado Egg Skillet**

   Prep time: 5 minutes | Cook time: 10 minutes | Serves 2

   How to serve and store: Serve hot, directly from the skillet. Store leftovers in an airtight container in the refrigerator for up to 2 days. Reheat in a skillet over medium heat until warmed through.

3. **Sausage Breakfast Stacks**

   Prep time: 10 minutes | Cook time: 15 minutes | Serves 2

   How to serve and store: Serve hot with freshly cracked black pepper on top. Store leftovers in an airtight container in the refrigerator for up to 3 days. Reheat in a skillet or microwave until warm.

4. **Turkey Reuben Sandwiches**

   Prep time: 5 minutes | Cook time: 15 minutes | Serves 4

   How to serve and store: Serve immediately while warm and toasty. Store leftovers in an airtight container in the refrigerator for up to 2 days. Reheat in a skillet until warmed through.

5. **Sticky Barbecued Ribs**

   Prep time: 10 minutes | Cook time: 1 hour 45 minutes | Serves 4

   How to serve and store: Serve hot, garnished with sesame seeds and chives. Store leftovers in an airtight container in the refrigerator for up to 3 days. Reheat in the oven at 300°F until heated through.

6. **Cheesy Edamame Spaghetti**

   Prep time: 5 minutes | Cook time: 10 minutes | Serves 4

   How to serve and store: Serve immediately, topped with the cashew mixture. Store leftovers in an airtight container in the refrigerator for up to 3 days. Reheat in the microwave or on the stove until warm.

7. **Vegetable Couscous with Peanut Sauce**

   Prep time: 5 minutes | Cook time: 10 minutes | Serves 2

   How to serve and store: Serve hot, drizzled with peanut sauce. Store leftovers in an airtight container in the refrigerator for up to 2 days. Reheat in the microwave before serving.

8. **Salted Peanut Butter Cookies**

   Prep time:10 minutes | Cook time: 40 minutes | Serves 4

   How to serve and store: Serve at room temperature or chilled. Store cookies carefully in an airtight container in the refrigerator for up to 5 days or in the freezer for up to 3 weeks.

9. **Chocolate-Avocado Pudding**

   Prep time: 5 minutes | Cook time: 10 minutes | Serves 3

   How to serve and store: Serve chilled. Store in an airtight container in the refrigerator for up to 2 days. Stir before serving if necessary.

WEEK 2 SHOPPING LIST

Pantry:

- Olive oil (5 tablespoons)
- Coconut flour (½ cup)
- Liquid stevia (4 teaspoons)
- Pink Himalayan salt (to taste)
- Freshly ground black pepper (to taste)
- Baking powder (3 teaspoons + 1 teaspoon)
- Granulated erythritol–monk fruit blend (1 cup)
- Swerve natural sweetener (1 tablespoon)
- Vanilla extract (¼ teaspoon)
- Kosher salt (to taste)
- Cayenne pepper (to taste)
- Stevia powder (½ teaspoon)
- American-style mustard (2 teaspoons)
- Granulated garlic (2 teaspoons)
- Garlic powder (1 teaspoon)

- Onion powder (½ teaspoon)
- Ground cumin powder (1 teaspoon)
- Ginger powder (1 teaspoon)
- Liquid smoke (2 teaspoons)
- Cocoa powder (4 tablespoons + 1 teaspoon)
- Almond flour, finely milled (1 cup)
- Rye bread (8 slices)
- Fat-free Thousand Island dressing (½ cup)
- Rice wine (2 tablespoons)

Grain:

- Couscous (1 cup)
- Brown rice spaghetti (4 ounces)

Fruit:

- Ripe banana (1)
- Avocado (3, sliced and mashed)
- Lemon juice (from 1 lemon)

Dairy:

- Cream cheese (10+2 ounces, room temperature)
- Swiss cheese (4 slices)
- Ghee (2 tablespoons)
- Butter (4 tablespoons + extra for coating and topping)
- Unsalted butter (8 tablespoons, room temperature)

Vegetables, Herbs, and Spices:

- Kale (5 ounces, sliced into ribbons)
- Sliced mushrooms (2 cups)
- Leek, sliced (1)
- Fresh parsley, finely chopped (2 cups)
- Fresh chives, chopped (4 tablespoons)
- Frozen mixed vegetables (2 cups, thawed)

- Sauerkraut, drained (1 cup)

Nuts and Seeds:

- Roasted cashews, unsalted (1 cup)
- Sesame seeds, toasted (2 tablespoons)
- All-natural peanut butter (1 cup, no added sugar)

Protein:

- Ground pork (8 ounces)
- Beef ribs (1 pound)
- Ground turkey (1 pound)
- Eggs (14 large)
- Sausage patties (2)
- Sliced turkey (6 ounces)

Legumes:

- Frozen edamame (3 cups, thawed)

WEEK 2 MEAL PREPARATION

To prepare for Pancake "Cake," start by preheating your oven to 425°F and coat a 9-by-13-inch baking pan with a generous amount of butter to prevent sticking. Next, in a food processor or blender, thoroughly combine the eggs, cream cheese, stevia, baking powder, and coconut flour into a smooth batter. If you'd like, you can mix in some additional ingredients for extra flavor. Then, spread 4 tablespoons of butter in the prepared pan before placing it in the oven for 2 to 3 minutes to allow the butter to melt. It's essential to watch the butter closely to ensure it doesn't brown or burn. After removing the pan from the oven, pour the batter into it and bake for approximately 15 minutes, or until a paring knife inserted into the center of the cake comes out clean. Once baked, transfer the cake to a cooling rack and add a few more tablespoons of melted butter on top if desired. Finally, cut the pancake "cake" into 4 servings and serve it while it's still warm.

While the cake is inside the oven, prepare the Kale-Avocado Egg Skillet. In a large skillet set over medium heat, gently heat 1 tablespoon of olive oil. Add the mushrooms to the pan and sauté for approximately 3 minutes until tender and golden. In a medium-sized bowl, lovingly massage the kale with the remaining 1 tablespoon of olive oil for 1 to 2 minutes to help tenderize it. Place the kale in the skillet on top of the mushrooms, and then delicately arrange the slices of avocado on top of the kale. With a spoon, carefully create 4 wells for the eggs. Gently crack one egg into each well. Generously season the eggs and kale with pink Himalayan salt and freshly ground pepper for added flavor. Cover the skillet and cook for about 5 minutes or until the eggs reach your preferred degree of doneness. Finally, serve this delectable dish while it's still hot.

Prepare for Sausage Breakfast Stacks while the kale-avocado egg is cooking. Start by preheating the oven to 375°F. In a medium-sized mixing bowl, thoroughly combine the ground pork, garlic powder, and onion powder, then shape the mixture into two patties. Next, heat 1 tablespoon of ghee in a medium skillet over medium-high heat and cook the sausage patties for 2 minutes on each side until they are nicely browned. Transfer the patties to a baking sheet and bake in the oven for 8 to 10 minutes until fully cooked. Add the remaining 1 tablespoon of ghee in the same skillet and fry the eggs without disturbing them for about 3 minutes until the whites are opaque and the yolks have set. Meanwhile, in a small bowl, mash the avocado. Season the eggs with pink Himalayan salt and pepper. Once the sausage patties are cooked, place each patty on a warmed plate, spread half of the mashed avocado on top of each patty, and place a fried egg on top.

While the sausages are cooking, prepare for Turkey Reuben Sandwiches. start by heating some oil in a nonstick skillet over medium heat. As the pan heats up, evenly divide the turkey, cheese, sauerkraut, and dressing between the slices of flavorful rye bread, creating two well-stacked sandwiches. Once the ingredients are in place, carefully place the sandwiches in the skillet and cook each side for about 3 minutes, until the bread turns golden brown and toasty while the cheese melts and the fillings warm up.

Prepare for Sticky Barbecued Ribs while the Turkey Reuben Sandwiches are cooking. Start by heating the olive oil in a large pan over a moderate flame. Once the oil is heated, carefully sear the beef ribs on each side for about 3 to 4 minutes until they develop a rich, caramelized crust. Then, add in the leeks and cook for 3 minutes until they soften and release their aroma. Now, it's time to deglaze the pan with a generous splash of wine, allowing the liquid to bubble and pick up all those wonderful browned bits from the bottom of the pan. Next, pour the remaining wine, broth, cumin powder, ginger powder, and a pinch of salt and pepper to season. Lower the heat to medium-low, cover the pan, and let it all simmer for a tantalizing 40 minutes, allowing the flavors to meld and the beef to become tender. Meanwhile, preheat the oven to 300 degrees F and line a baking dish with foil. Once the meat is ready, carefully transfer the ribs and cooking liquid to the prepared baking dish. Drizzle with a touch of liquid smoke, add minced garlic, a hint of stevia for sweetness, and a dollop of American-style mustard for a subtle tang. Place the baking dish in the oven and let the ribs bake for about an hour, turning them occasionally to ensure they are evenly coated with the flavorful glaze. Once done, sprinkle the ribs with sesame seeds and freshly chopped chives for a fragrant, fresh finish.

While the ribs are inside the oven, prepare for Cheesy Edamame Spaghetti. Start by filling a large pot with water and bringing it to a boil over high heat. Once the water is boiling, add the pasta and let it cook for about 10 minutes or until it's al dente. After draining the pasta and transferring it to a bowl, you can then prepare the cashew topping by combining cashews, cheese, garlic powder, and salt in a food processor. Pulse the ingredients until a coarse texture is achieved and set it aside. Toss the cooked pasta with edamame, parsley, oil, and pepper to finish. Top it with the cashew mixture, toss to combine, and then it's ready to serve.

Prepare for Vegetable Couscous with Peanut Sauce while the spaghetti is cooking. Start by bringing the water and butter to a boil over high heat in a medium saucepan. Once the mixture reaches a rolling boil, remove the pan from the heat and gently stir in the couscous and a pinch of salt. Cover the saucepan and let it sit for 15 minutes, allowing the couscous to absorb the liquid and become fluffy. Then, mix in a colorful assortment of fresh vegetables to add vibrancy and nutrients to the couscous. Generously drizzle the dish with an irresistible Easy Peanut Sauce to elevate it. Finally, serve this flavorful and wholesome couscous dish promptly to enjoy the delightful combination of textures and flavors.

While the water is boiling, prepare for Salted Peanut Butter Cookies. Preheat your oven to 350°F and line a baking sheet with parchment paper. In a large bowl, use a medium-high speed electric mixer to blend the peanut butter, erythritol-monk fruit blend, butter, and egg until well combined, scraping the bowl as needed. Add the almond flour and baking powder, and mix on low until fully incorporated. Use a small cookie scoop or spoon to portion the dough onto the prepared baking sheet, then flatten each cookie with a fork to create a crisscross pattern. Sprinkle the tops with salt before baking for 10 to 12 minutes or until the edges turn lightly brown. Allow the cookies to cool completely before enjoying them. Handle the cookies carefully when storing them, as they can be delicate. Store them in the refrigerator for up to 5 days or in the freezer for up to 3 weeks.

Prepare for Chocolate Avocado Pudding while the Salted Peanut Butter Cookies are baking. Start by combining ripe avocado, smooth cream cheese, a touch of sweetener, rich cocoa powder, fragrant vanilla extract, and a pinch of pink Himalayan salt in a food processor or blender. Blend the ingredients until they are entirely smooth and free of any lumps. Once the mousse is ready, carefully transfer it into two small dessert bowls and allow it to chill in the refrigerator for at least 30 minutes before serving.

MEAL PLAN WEEK 3

1. **Pb & Banana French Toast**

   Prep time: **10 minutes** |Cook time: **10 minutes**| Serves **2**

   How to serve and store: Serve warm with Greek yogurt. Store leftovers in an airtight container in the refrigerator for up to 2 days. Reheat in a skillet before serving.

2. **Mushroom-Feta Egg Cups**

   Prep time: **10 minutes** |Cook time: **20 minutes**| Serves **4**

   How to serve and store: Serve immediately with peanut butter toast. Store egg cups in an airtight container in the refrigerator for up to 4 days. Reheat in the microwave.

3. **Bacon and Egg Cauliflower Hash**

   Prep time: **5 minutes** | Cook time: **15 minutes** | Serves **2**

   How to serve and store: Serve hot. Store leftovers in an airtight container in the refrigerator for up to 3 days. Reheat in a skillet over medium heat.

4. **Chicken with Mango Salsa**

   Prep time: **10 minutes** |Cook time: **25 minutes**| Serves **4**

   How to serve and store: Serve chicken topped with mango salsa on mixed greens. Store leftovers separately in airtight containers in the refrigerator for up to 3 days.

5. **Crispy Mexican Pork Carnitas**

   Prep time: **5 minutes** | Cook time: **45 minutes** |Serves **4**

   How to serve and store: Serve hot. Store in an airtight container in the refrigerator for up to 4 days. Reheat in a skillet until warmed through.

6. **Shrimp Scampi with Whole Wheat Pasta**

   Prep time: **15 minutes** | Cook time: **20 minutes** | Serves **4**

   How to serve and store: Serve immediately. Store leftovers in an airtight container in the refrigerator for up to 3 days. Reheat gently in a skillet.

7. **Fish Taco Bowl**

   Prep time: **10 minutes** | Cook time: **15 minutes** | Serves **2**

   How to serve and store: Serve warm with a drizzle of mayo sauce. Store components separately in airtight containers in the refrigerator for up to 2 days.

8. **Protein Cheesecake**

   Prep time: **5 minutes** | Cook time: **10 minutes** | Serves **12**

   How to serve and store: Serve chilled. Store in the refrigerator, covered, for up to 5 days. Freeze individual slices for up to 2 months.

9. **Chocolate-Dipped Peanut Butter Ice Pops**

   Prep time:**10 minutes** | Cook time:**5 minutes** | Serves **12**

How to serve and store: Serve frozen. Store in an airtight container in the freezer for up to 3 weeks.

WEEK 3 SHOPPING LIST

Pantry:

- Ground cinnamon (½ teaspoon + ⅛ teaspoon)
- Vanilla extract (1 ½ teaspoons)
- Nonstick cooking spray
- Pink Himalayan salt
- Freshly ground black pepper
- Sea salt
- Olive oil (3 tablespoons + more for cooking)
- Dijon mustard (2 tablespoons)
- Tomato ketchup (2 tablespoons)
- Tajín seasoning salt (4 teaspoons)
- Spicy Red Pepper Miso Mayo (1 tablespoon + more for serving)
- Stevia (¾ cup)
- Granulated erythritol–monk fruit blend (¼ cup or 2 tablespoons)
- Semisweet chocolate chips (2 tablespoons)
- Sugar-free chocolate chips (4 ounces)
- Coconut oil (2 tablespoons)

Grain:

- 100% whole-grain bread (12 slices)
- Whole wheat pasta (½ pound)

Dairy:

- Nonfat plain Greek yogurt (1 cup)
- Low-fat feta cheese (½ cup, crumbled)
- Fat-free cream cheese (24 ounces)
- Full-fat cream cheese (8 ounces)
- Heavy (whipping) cream (2 cups)

Fruit:

- Small banana (1)
- Avocado (2)
- Fresh or frozen mango (1 cup, diced)
- Lime juice (2 tablespoons)
- Vegetables, Herbs, and Spices:
- Cherry tomatoes (2 cups, halved)
- White button mushrooms (2 cups, chopped)
- Scallions (6, green parts only, chopped)
- Cauliflower (½ head, cut into small florets)
- Garlic cloves (5, minced)
- Medium onion (1, diced)
- Mixed greens (8 cups)
- Red onion (¼ cup, minced)
- Coleslaw cabbage mix (2 cups)

Nuts and Seeds:

- 100% all-natural peanut butter (4 tablespoons + 1 cup)

Protein:

- Large eggs (18)
- Large egg whites (8)
- Boneless, skinless chicken breasts (4, 4-ounce each)
- Pork butt (2 pounds, cut into 2-inch cubes)
- Large shrimp (1 pound, peeled and deveined)
- Tilapia fillets (2, 5-ounce each)
- Protein powder, vanilla (½ cup)

WEEK 3 MEAL PREPARATION

To prepare for Pb & Banana French Toast In a shallow bowl, whisk together the eggs, ½ teaspoon of cinnamon, and a splash of vanilla until well combined. Set the mixture aside. Take 2 slices of bread and spread 1 tablespoon of creamy peanut butter on each slice. Arrange half of the banana slices on one of them and then place the other slice over it to form a sandwich. Repeat the process with the remaining 2 slices of bread. Next, heat a skillet over medium heat and lightly coat it with nonstick cooking spray. Dip each sandwich into the egg mixture, ensuring both sides are well soaked, before placing it onto the skillet. Cook the sandwiches until they turn golden brown, taking 2 to 4 minutes on each side. Once cooked, sprinkle the sandwiches with the remaining ⅛ teaspoon of cinnamon and serve them with a dollop of Greek yogurt on the side.

While the banana french toast is cooking, prepare for Mushroom-Feta Egg Cups. Preheat the oven to 350°F. Lightly spray a 12-cup muffin tin with nonstick cooking spray. Next, evenly distribute the tomatoes, mushrooms, and scallions among the muffin cups. Sprinkle each with feta and then pour the egg whites over the vegetables, ensuring each cup has an equal portion—season with salt and pepper to taste. Place the muffin tin in the oven and bake for approximately 20 minutes or until the egg is fully set. Once done, carefully remove the egg cups from the muffin tin and arrange 3 cups on each of 4 plates. Meanwhile, spread the peanut butter evenly on the slices of toast and place 2 slices on each plate.

Prepare for Bacon and Egg Cauliflower Hash while the Mushroom-Feta Egg Cups are baking. In a large skillet placed over medium-high heat, carefully cook the bacon on both sides until it turns crispy, which should take around 8 minutes. Then, transfer the bacon to a plate lined with paper towels to drain and cool for about 5

minutes. Once cooled, transfer the bacon to a cutting board and chop it. Next, adjust the heat to medium and add the cauliflower, garlic, and onion to the leftover bacon grease in the skillet. Sauté this delicious combination for approximately 5 minutes. If the pan starts to get dry, feel free to add some olive oil. The goal is to achieve a tender-crisp texture for the cauliflower florets just before adding the eggs. With a spoon, create 4 wells in the skillet mixture and carefully crack an egg into each well. Proceed to season the eggs and hash with pink Himalayan salt and pepper, enhancing the flavor profile. Allow the eggs to cook until they set, which should take around 3 minutes. To finish, sprinkle the diced bacon over the hash mixture, adding a final touch of flavor, and serve the dish while it's still hot and delightful.

While the bacon and egg cauliflower cook, prepare for Chicken with Mango Salsa. start by preheating the oven to 400°F and lining a baking sheet with aluminum foil. Next, use a basting brush to generously spread olive oil over the chicken and season it with a pinch of salt and freshly ground black pepper. Arrange the seasoned chicken on the prepared baking sheet and let it bake for 20 to 25 minutes or until it is perfectly cooked. While the chicken is baking, take a large bowl and mix the ripe avocado, sweet mango, minced garlic, finely diced red onion, and freshly chopped cilantro. Add the juice of a lime and a drizzle of oil to the mixture, stirring until everything is thoroughly combined. Cover the bowl with plastic wrap and refrigerate the flavorful mango salsa until ready to serve. When the chicken is done, plate a tender chicken breast on each of 4 plates. Divide a generous portion of mixed greens between the plates and top them with the refreshing mango salsa.

Prepare for Crispy Mexican Pork Carnitas while the Chicken with Mango Salsa is cooking.

Start by greasing a stockpot or Dutch oven with nonstick cooking spray. Heat the pot over medium-high heat and sear the pork butt until it turns a rich, golden brown and is thoroughly cooked. Once the pork is browned, carefully incorporate the remaining ingredients into the stockpot, ensuring everything is well combined. Next, transfer the flavorful mixture to a baking dish, cover it with foil, and place it in a preheated oven set to 350 degrees F for approximately 35 minutes. After baking, switch the oven to broil and cook the meat for about 7 minutes or until the top develops a delectably crisp texture. Once it's done, serve the dish immediately.

While the pork cooks, prepare for Shrimp Scampi with Whole Wheat Pasta. Begin by cooking the pasta to perfection according to the instructions on the package. Meanwhile, heat up a generous amount of olive oil in a large skillet over medium-high heat. Once the oil is sizzling, add the shrimp and cook them for 2-3 minutes on each side until they turn a delightful shade of pink and are cooked through. Set the shrimp aside once they are done. In the same skillet, infuse the air with the irresistible aroma of garlic as it sizzles for a minute. Then, elevate the dish by deglazing the skillet with white wine and a splash of lemon juice. Watch as the sauce comes to life, thickening and becoming irresistible as it simmers for 2-3 minutes. Finally, combine the tantalizing sauce with the cooked pasta and shrimp, ensuring each strand is coated in a rich, flavorful sauce. Sprinkle with fresh parsley to add a pop of color and freshness, and serve immediately.

Prepare for a Fish Taco Bowl while the Shrimp Scampi with Whole Wheat Pasta is cooking. Preheat your oven to 425°F and prepare a baking sheet by lining it with aluminum foil or a silicone baking mat. Begin by gently massaging some olive oil onto the tilapia, then generously coat it with 2 teaspoons of flavorful Tajín seasoning salt. Place the seasoned fish on the prepared pan and let it bake for about 15 minutes or until it reaches an opaque consistency when pierced with a fork. Once done, transfer the fish to a cooling rack and rest for 4 minutes. In the meantime, delicately combine the coleslaw with a mayo-based sauce in a medium bowl, ensuring the cabbage is lightly dressed. Introduce some mashed avocado and the remaining 2 teaspoons of Tajín seasoning salt to the coleslaw, and season with a sprinkle of pink Himalayan salt and black pepper. Divide this delectable salad between two bowls. Using two forks, shred the baked fish into bite-sized pieces and add them to the bowls. Finish by drizzling more of the mayo sauce over the fish before serving.

While the fish taco bowl is cooking, prepare for Protein Cheesecake. Start by preheating your oven to 350°F and spraying a 9" pie pan with nonstick cooking spray. In a large bowl, combine cream cheese, protein powder, stevia, vanilla, eggs, and lemon juice, then mix with a hand mixer on medium speed until smooth. Next, sprinkle the mixture into the prepared pan with chocolate chips. Bake the cheesecake for 45 minutes, remove it from the oven, and let it cool on a rack for 1 hour. After cooling, refrigerate the cheesecake for at least 3 hours before serving for the best results.

Prepare for Chocolate-Dipped Peanut Butter Ice Pops while the protein cheesecake is inside the oven. Use a medium-high electric mixer in a large bowl to beat the cream cheese, peanut butter, confectioners' erythritol–monk fruit blend, vanilla, and salt until smooth. Add the heavy cream and mix until well combined. Pour the mixture into popsicle molds, insert the sticks, and freeze for 3 to 4 hours until completely frozen. Meanwhile, melt the chocolate baking chips and coconut oil in a microwave-safe bowl in 30-second intervals, and let it cool for 5 to 10 minutes. Line a baking sheet with parchment paper. Once the popsicles are frozen, dip them halfway into the melted chocolate, place them on the prepared sheet, and return them to the freezer for about 20 minutes. Store the chocolate-dipped popsicles in the freezer in an airtight (non-glass) container for up to 3 weeks. Enjoy!

MEAL PLAN WEEK 4

1. Avocado and Eggs

Prep time: 10 minutes | Cook time: 20 minutes | Serves 4

How to serve and store: Serve warm with a sprinkle of fresh herbs. Store leftovers in an airtight container in the fridge for up to 2 days. Reheat in the oven at 350°F for 5-7 minutes.

2. Nut and Berry Breakfast Bowl

Prep time: 5 minutes, plus 10 minutes to stand | Cook time: 15 minutes | Serves 2

How to serve and store: Serve cold, topped with fresh berries. Store in the refrigerator for up to 3 days. Stir before eating.

3. Rosemary & Thyme Flat Bread

Prep time: 15 minutes | Cook time: 20 minutes | Serves 3

How to serve and store: Serve warm as a side or snack. Store in an airtight container at room temperature for up to 2 days or in the fridge for up to 4 days. Reheat in a skillet or oven.

4. Bacon & Cheese Chicken

Prep time: 30 minutes | Cook time: 19 minutes | Serves 4

How to serve and store: Serve hot with a side of veggies or salad. Store in an airtight container in the fridge for up to 3 days. Reheat in the oven at 350°F until warm.

5. Thai Ground Beef Curry

Prep time: 10 minutes | Cook time: 35 minutes |Serves 6

How to serve and store: Serve hot over rice or cauliflower rice. Store in the fridge for up to 4 days or freeze for up to 2 months. Reheat on the stovetop or microwave.

6. Tilapia with Olives & Tomato Sauce

Prep time: 30 minutes | Cook time: 38 minutes | Serves 4

How to serve and store: Serve warm with a side of steamed vegetables. Store in an airtight container in the fridge for up to 3 days. Reheat gently on the stovetop.

7. **Eggplant Pizzas**

   Prep time: 5 minutes | Cook time: 10 minutes | Serves 4

   How to serve and store: Serve warm, topped with fresh basil. Store in an airtight container in the fridge for up to 2 days. Reheat under the broiler for 3-4 minutes.

8. **No-Bake Pumpkin Protein Bars**

   Prep time: 5 minutes | Cook time: 10 minutes | Serves 8

   How to serve and store: Serve chilled or at room temperature. Store in the refrigerator for up to 1 week or freeze for up to 2 months. Thaw overnight in the fridge if frozen.

9. **Cookie Fat Bombs**

   Prep time: 10 minutes | Cook time: 15 minutes | Serves 6

   How to serve and store: Serve cold or at room temperature. Store in the fridge for up to 1 week or in the freezer for up to 2 months. Enjoy straight from the fridge or let sit at room temperature for a few minutes if frozen.

WEEK 4 SHOPPING LIST

Pantry:

- Almond flour (½ cup)
- Gluten-free baking powder (1 ½ teaspoons)
- Unsweetened almond butter (1 tablespoon + ½ cup)
- Coconut flour (½ cup)
- Vanilla protein powder (¼ cup)

- Pumpkin pie spice (¾ teaspoon)
- Maple syrup (1/3 cup)
- Vanilla extract (1 teaspoon)
- Cacao nibs or vegan keto chocolate chips (¼ cup + ½ cup)
- Coconut aminos (1 ounce)
- Ranch dressing (1 ounce)
- Sea salt
- Freshly ground black pepper
- Ground turmeric (¼ teaspoon)
- Ginger-garlic paste (1 teaspoon)
- Red curry paste (1 teaspoon)
- Cumin (½ teaspoon)
- Salt (½ teaspoon)
- Pepper (1/3 teaspoon)
- Garlic powder (1 teaspoon)
- Tallow (2 teaspoons)
- Olive oil (3 tablespoons + extra for cooking)
- Coconut oil (1 tablespoon)
- Tomato sauce (1 ½ cups)
- Semisweet chocolate chips (½ cup)

Grain:

- Rolled oats (2 tablespoons)

Fruit:

- Avocados (2)
- Blueberries (⅓ cup)
- Raspberries (⅓ cup)
- Canned pumpkin purée (½ cup)

Dairy:

- Cheddar cheese (¼ cup)
- Monterey Jack cheese (4 ounces, grated)
- Part-skim mozzarella cheese (4 ounces, thinly sliced)

- Unsweetened almond milk (1 cup)

Vegetables, Herbs, and Spices:

- Green onions (chopped)
- Fresh thyme (2 teaspoons, chopped)
- Fresh rosemary (3 tablespoons, chopped)
- Garlic cloves (2, minced)
- Oregano (1 teaspoon)
- Red onion (½, chopped)
- Parsley (1 tablespoon)
- Kalamata olives (¼ cup)
- Italian seasoning (½ teaspoon)
- Red curry paste (1 teaspoon)

Nuts and Seeds:

- Raw pumpkin seeds (2 tablespoons)
- Chia seeds (2 tablespoons)
- Hemp hearts (2 tablespoons)
- Walnuts (2 tablespoons)

Protein:

- Large eggs (4)
- Chicken breast (1 (4-ounce), cooked and shredded)
- Chicken breasts (4)
- Ground chuck (1 ½ pounds)
- Tilapia fillets (4)

WEEK 4 MEAL PREPARATION

To prepare for Avocados and Eggs, preheat your oven to 425°F and take ripe avocado halves. Using a spoon, carefully hollow each side until the hole is about twice the original size. Place the prepared avocado halves in an 8-by-8-inch baking dish, ensuring they are hollow-side up. Then, crack an egg into each hollow, creating a perfect nest.

After that, divide some flavorful shredded chicken between each avocado half, adding a delightful protein-rich touch. To elevate the dish further, sprinkle a generous amount of cheese on top of each avocado half, ensuring every bite is filled with rich, savory flavors. To enhance the taste profile, season lightly with salt and pepper, perfectly complementing the natural creaminess of the avocado. Now, carefully place the baking dish in the oven and bake the avocados until the eggs are cooked, typically taking 15 to 20 minutes.

While the avocado and eggs cook, prepare for the Nut and Berry Breakfast Bowl. Combine the almond milk, pumpkin seeds, chia seeds, hemp hearts, walnuts, and oats in a medium bowl. Let the mixture sit on the counter for 10 minutes to thicken, then stir in the almond butter. Divide the soaked mixture between two storage containers and top each with a portion of blueberries and raspberries before sealing the containers.

Prepare for Rosemary & Thyme flatbread while the nut and berry breakfast bowl cooks. start by combining all the ingredients except olive oil in a blender or food processor, and blend until well combined. Then, heat one-third of the olive oil in a large frying pan over medium heat. Pour one-third of the mixture into the frying pan and cook for about 3 minutes or until bubbles appear. Carefully flip the flatbread and continue cooking for an additional 3 minutes. Once done, remove the flatbread from the pan and repeat the process with the remaining batter.

While the flatbread is cooking, prepare for Bacon & Cheese Chicken. Heat some oil over high heat and cook the chicken breasts for 7 minutes on each side. In another pan over medium heat, cook the bacon until crispy, then crumble it. Transfer the chicken to a baking dish and add green onions, coconut aminos, cheese, and crumbled bacon. Place the dish in the oven, turn on the broiler, and cook for 5 minutes at high temperature. Once done, divide the chicken among serving plates.

Prepare for Thai Ground Beef Curry while the bacon and cheese chicken is cooking. In a deep saucepan, start by melting the tallow over medium heat. Once the tallow is hot, add the ground meat and brown it for 5 to 6 minutes, making sure to crumble it with a fork as it cooks. Next, add the remaining ingredients to the saucepan and stir everything together. Reduce the heat to low and let the mixture simmer, partially covered, for about 25 minutes. Ensure the meat is thoroughly cooked before ladling the dish into individual bowls. Serve the warm.

While the Thai ground beef curry is cooking, prepare for Tilapia with Olives & Tomato Sauce. start by heating olive oil in a skillet over medium heat and sautéing the onion for 3 minutes. Then, add minced garlic and oregano, and cook for 30 seconds to release their flavors. Next, stir in the tomatoes and bring the mixture to a gentle boil. Reduce the heat and let it simmer for 5 minutes to allow the flavors to meld together. Then, add pitted olives and the tilapia fillets to the skillet and cook for about 8 minutes or until the fish is cooked through. Finally, serve the tilapia with the flavorful tomato sauce.

Prepare for Eggplant Pizzas while the tilapia is cooking. Start by preheating the broiler and lining a baking sheet with parchment paper. Brush each side of the eggplant slices with oil and season them with salt and pepper. Next, heat a large nonstick skillet over medium heat and cook the eggplant slices in batches until tender and lightly browned, which should take about 3 to 5 minutes per side. Once cooked, transfer the eggplant slices to the prepared baking sheet and top each one with tomato sauce, Italian seasoning, and cheese. Then, broil the eggplant for 3 to 5 minutes or until the cheese is melted and lightly browned. Finally, top the broiled eggplant with fresh basil and serve

While the eggplant pizza is cooking, prepare for No-Bake Pumpkin Protein Bars. Start by lining an 8" × 8" baking pan with parchment paper. Mix coconut flour, protein powder, and pumpkin pie spice in a large bowl. In a small saucepan, heat almond butter, maple syrup, and vanilla over low heat until melted and combined, then add this to the flour mixture along with pumpkin and milk. Stir everything together until well combined, then fold in some chocolate chips. The dough will be thick. Transfer the dough to the prepared pan and press it firmly with a spatula to pack it evenly. Refrigerate for at least 30 minutes, then slice into eight bars and serve.

Prepare for Cookie Fat Bombs while the protein bars are baking. start by lining a baking sheet with parchment paper. You can use aluminum foil or a greased pan if you don't have parchment paper. Whisk together the almond butter, coconut flour, and cinnamon in a mixing bowl, and then fold in the cacao nibs. After mixing the ingredients, cover the bowl and place it in the freezer for 15 to 20 minutes. Once chilled, remove the bowl from the freezer and use a spoon or a cookie scoop to form the mixture into small balls by rolling it between your palms. Place the fat bomb balls on the prepared baking sheet and return them to the freezer to chill for about 20 minutes or until firm.

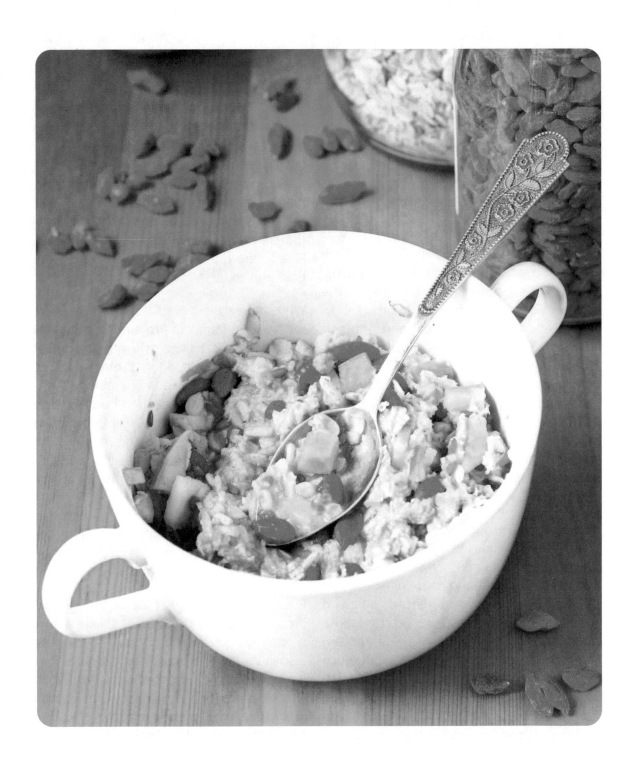

CHAPTER 3:
BREAKFAST

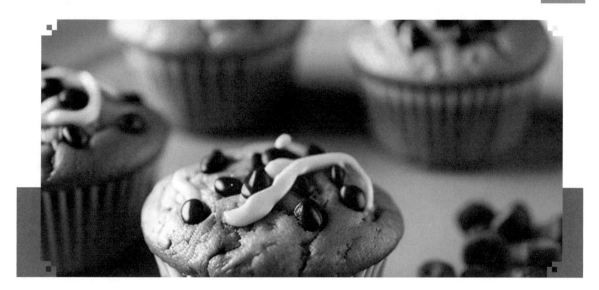

ROSEMARY & THYME FLAT BREAD

Prep time: 15 minutes | Cook time: 20 minutes | Serves 3

- ½ cup almond flour
- 8 large egg whites
- 1 ½ teaspoon gluten-free baking powder
- 2 teaspoons fresh thyme, chopped
- ¼ teaspoon ground turmeric
- 3 tablespoons fresh rosemary, chopped
- 2 tablespoons olive oil
- ¼ teaspoon salt

1. In a blender or food processor, combine all of the ingredients except for the olive oil and blend until well combined.
2. In a large frying pan, heat about a third of the olive oil over medium heat.
3. Pour one-third of the mixture into the frying pan and allow to cook for about 3 minutes until bubbles start to appear. Flip carefully and continue cooking for an additional 3 minutes.
4. Remove the flatbread from the pan and repeat with the remaining batter.

Per Serving

Calories: **300** | Carbs: **10g** | Fiber: **5g** | Fat: **23g** | Protein: **16g**

PEANUT BUTTER AND BANANA MUG MUFFINS

Prep time: 5 minutes | Cook time: 5 minutes | Serves 3

- nonstick cooking spray
- 1 ripe banana, mashed
- ¾ cup egg whites
- ¾ cup quick oats
- 3 tablespoons peanut butter
- 1½ teaspoons vanilla extract
- 1½ teaspoons ground cinnamon
- 3 tablespoons mini chocolate chips (optional)

1. Spray 3 large mugs with nonstick cooking spray.
2. In a medium bowl, combine the banana, egg whites, oats, peanut butter, vanilla, and cinnamon. Mix well, then fold in the chocolate chips (if using).
3. Divide the batter equally among the 3 mugs.
4. Microwave each mug on high for 2 minutes, or until the muffin is cooked through and the top is firm to the touch.
5. Remove from the microwave. Free the sides of the muffins from the mugs with a butter knife, and turn the mugs upside down to shake onto a plate. Let cool.
6. Into each of 3 airtight storage containers, place 1 muffin and seal.

Per Serving

Calories: **325** | Fat: **15g** | Protein: **15g** | Carbs: **35g** |Fiber: **6g**

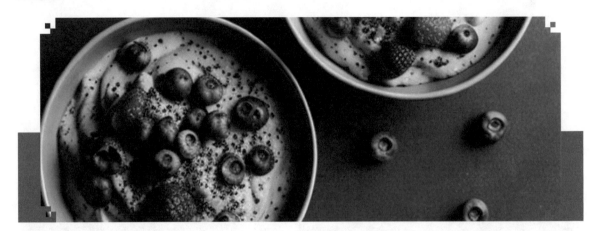

NUT AND BERRY BREAKFAST BOWL

Prep time: **5 minutes, plus 10 minutes to stand | Cook time: 15 minutes | Serves 2**

- 1 cup unsweetened vanilla almond milk
- 2 tablespoons raw pumpkin seeds
- 2 tablespoons chia seeds
- 2 tablespoons hemp hearts
- 2 tablespoons walnuts
- 2 tablespoons rolled oats
- 1 tablespoon unsweetened almond butter
- ⅓ cup blueberries
- ⅓ cup raspberries

1. In a medium bowl, mix together the almond milk, pumpkin seeds, chia seeds, hemp hearts, walnuts, and oats.
2. Let sit on the counter to thicken for 10 minutes. Stir in the almond butter.
3. Into each of 2 storage containers, place half of the soaked mixture. Top each with half of the blueberries and raspberries and seal.

Per Serving

Calories: 317 | Fat: 22g | Protein: 12g | Carbs: 21g | Fiber: 10g

SAUSAGE BREAKFAST STACKS

Prep time: **10 minutes | Cook time: 15 minutes | Serves 2**

- 8 ounces ground pork
- ½ teaspoon garlic powder
- ½ teaspoon onion powder
- 2 tablespoons
- ghee, divided
- 2 large eggs
- 1 avocado
- Pink Himalayan salt
- Freshly ground black pepper

1. Preheat the oven to 375°F.
2. In a medium bowl, mix well to combine the ground pork, garlic powder, and onion powder. Form the mixture into 2 patties.
3. In a medium skillet over medium-high heat, melt 1 tablespoon of ghee.
4. Add the sausage patties and cook for 2 minutes on each side, until browned.
5. Transfer the sausage to a baking sheet. Cook in the oven for 8 to 10 minutes, until cooked through.
6. Add the remaining 1 tablespoon of ghee to the skillet. When it is hot, crack the eggs into the skillet and cook without disturbing for about 3 minutes, until the whites are opaque and the yolks have set.
7. Meanwhile, in a small bowl, mash the avocado.
8. Season the eggs with pink Himalayan salt and pepper.
9. Remove the cooked sausage patties from the oven.
10. Place a sausage patty on each of two warmed plates. Spread half of the mashed avocado on top of each sausage patty, and top each with a fried egg. Serve hot.

Per Serving

Calories: 533 | Fat: 44g | Carbs: 7g | Fiber: 5g | Protein: 29g

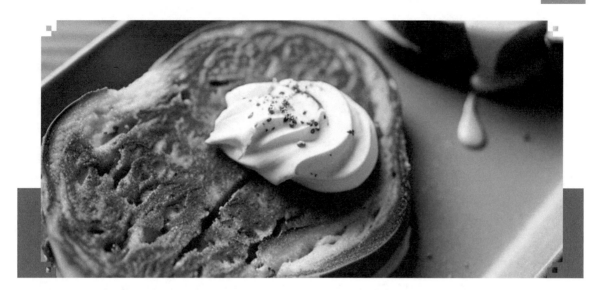

MUSHROOM-FETA EGG CUPS

Prep time: 10 minutes |**Cook time: 20 minutes**| **Serves 4**

- Nonstick cooking spray
- 2 cups halved cherry tomatoes
- 2 cups chopped white button mushrooms
- 6 scallions, green parts only, chopped
- ½ cup crumbled low-fat feta cheese
- 8 large egg whites, plus 4 whole large eggs, beaten
- Sea salt
- Freshly ground black pepper
- 2 tablespoons creamy 100% all-natural peanut butter
- 8 slices 100% whole-grain bread, lightly toasted

1. Preheat the oven to 350°F. Lightly spray 12-cup muffin tin with nonstick cooking spray.
2. Divide the tomatoes, mushrooms, and scallions equally in the 12 muffin cups. Top each with the feta. Pour the egg whites equally over the vegetables. Season with salt and pepper.
3. Bake for 20 minutes, or until the egg is set. Remove the egg cups from the muffin tin and place 3 on each of 4 plates. Spread the peanut butter equally on the slices of toast and place 2 on each plate. Serve immediately.

Per Serving

Calories: 299| **Fat: 11g**| **Carbs: 31g**|**Fiber: 6g**| **Protein: 21g**

PB & BANANA FRENCH TOAST

Prep time: 10 minutes |**Cook time: 10 minutes**| **Serves 2**

- 2 large eggs
- ½ teaspoon plus ⅛ teaspoon ground cinnamon, divided
- ¼ teaspoon vanilla extract
- 2 tablespoons creamy 100% all-natural peanut
- butter, divided
- 4 slices 100% whole-grain bread
- 1 small banana, cut into slices
- Nonstick cooking spray
- 1 cup nonfat plain Greek yogurt

1. In a shallow bowl, beat together the eggs, ½ teaspoon of cinnamon, and vanilla. Set aside.
2. Spread 1 tablespoon peanut butter on 1 slice of bread, top with half of the banana slices, and close with the second slice of bread to make a sandwich. Repeat with the remaining 2 slices of bread.
3. Lightly spray a skillet with nonstick cooking spray and set over medium heat.
4. Carefully soak both sides of the sandwich in the egg mixture. Cook the sandwich in a skillet until golden brown, 2 to 4 minutes on each side. Repeat with the remaining sandwich.
5. Sprinkle the sandwiches with the remaining ⅛ teaspoon cinnamon and serve with the Greek yogurt.

Per Serving

Calories: 430| **Fat: 16g**| **Carbs: 42g**|**Fiber: 7g**| **Protein: 31g**

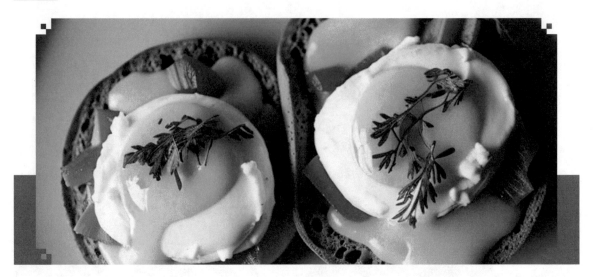

KALE-AVOCADO EGG SKILLET

Prep time: 5 minutes | **Cook time:** 10 minutes | Serves 2

- 2 tablespoons olive oil, divided
- 2 cups sliced mushrooms
- 5 ounces fresh kale, stemmed and sliced into ribbons
- 1 avocado, sliced
- 4 large eggs
- Pink Himalayan salt
- Freshly ground black pepper

1. In a large skillet over medium heat, heat 1 tablespoon of olive oil.
2. Add the mushrooms to the pan, and sauté for about 3 minutes.
3. In a medium bowl, massage the kale with the remaining 1 tablespoon of olive oil for 1 to 2 minutes to help tenderize it. Add the kale to the skillet on top of the mushrooms, then place the slices of avocado on top of the kale.
4. Using a spoon, create 4 wells for the eggs. Crack one egg into each well. Season the eggs and kale with pink Himalayan salt and pepper.
5. Cover the skillet and cook for about 5 minutes, or until the eggs reach your desired degree of doneness.
6. Serve hot.

Per Serving

Calories: 407 | **Fat:** 34g | **Carbs:** 13g | **Fiber:** 7g | **Protein:** 18g

EASY EGGS BENEDICT

Prep time: 10 minutes | **Cook time:** 15 minutes | Serves 4

- 2 large egg yolks
- ½ cup (1 stick) unsalted butter, melted but not hot
- 1 teaspoon lemon juice
- ½ teaspoon distilled white vinegar
- ½ teaspoon pink Himalayan salt
- 2 large eggs
- 1 tablespoon distilled white vinegar
- 1 English Muffin
- 2 slices Canadian bacon, cooked

1. Put all the ingredients for the hollandaise in a tall, narrow cup that is wide enough to fit an immersion blender and blend until smooth. Set aside.
2. Fill a saucepan halfway full of water. Add the vinegar and bring to a simmer over medium heat.
3. Crack each egg into a small ramekin and set aside. Once the water reaches a simmer, use a spoon to quickly swirl the water in one direction until it's spinning like a whirlpool.
4. Drop an egg into the center of the whirlpool and cook for 3 to 5 minutes, until the white is fully cooked. Remove with a slotted spoon and immediately place in an ice bath. Repeat the process with the second egg.
5. To assemble, slice the muffin in half and toast in a toaster or in the oven. Lay the halves on a plate. Top each half with a slice of Canadian bacon and a poached egg. Drizzle on one-quarter of the hollandaise sauce. Serve immediately.

Per Serving

Calories: 651 | **Fat:** 54.8 g | **Protein:** 26.3 g | **Carbs:** 14.4g | **Fiber:** 9.5 g

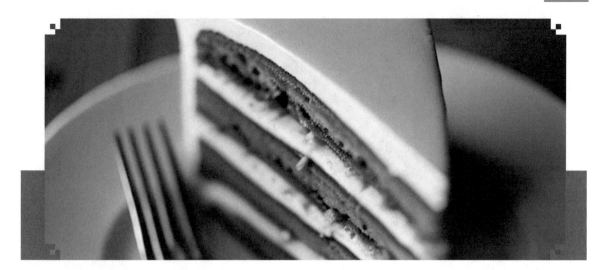

BACON AND EGG CAULIFLOWER HASH

Prep time: 5 minutes | **Cook time:** 15 minutes | Serves 2

- 6 bacon slices
- ½ head cauliflower, cut into small florets
- 2 garlic cloves, minced
- 1 medium onion, diced
- 4 large eggs
- 1 tablespoon olive oil, if needed
- Pink Himalayan salt
- Freshly ground black pepper

1. In a large skillet over medium-high heat, cook the bacon on both sides until crispy, about 8 minutes. Transfer the bacon to a paper towel–lined plate to drain and cool for 5 minutes. Transfer to a cutting board, and chop the bacon.
2. Turn the heat down to medium, and add the cauliflower, garlic, and onion to the bacon grease in the skillet. Sauté for 5 minutes. If the pan gets dry, add the olive oil. You want the cauliflower florets to just begin to brown before you add the eggs.
3. Using a spoon, make 4 wells in the mixture in the skillet, and crack an egg into each well. Season the eggs and hash with pink Himalayan salt and pepper. Cook the eggs until they set, about 3 minutes.
4. Sprinkle the diced bacon onto the hash mixture, and serve hot.

Per Serving

Calories: **395** | Fat: **27g** | Carbs: **15g** | Fiber: **4g** | Protein: **25g**

PANCAKE "CAKE"

Prep time: 5 minutes | **Cook time:** 20 minutes | Serves 4

- 4 tablespoons butter, plus more for the pan and the top of the cake
- 8 large eggs
- 8 ounces cream cheese, at room temperature
- 4 teaspoons liquid stevia
- 3 teaspoons baking powder
- ½ cup coconut flour

1. Preheat the oven to 425°F. Coat a 9-by-13-inch baking pan with butter.
2. In a food processor (or blender), process the eggs, cream cheese, stevia, baking powder, and coconut flour until thoroughly combined.
3. Mix in some add-ins (see Variations), if desired.
4. Spread out the 4 tablespoons of butter in the prepared pan.
5. Put the pan in the oven for 2 to 3 minutes to melt the butter. Let the butter bubble, but make sure it doesn't brown or burn. Remove from the oven.
6. Pour the batter into the pan.
7. Bake for about 15 minutes, or until a paring knife stuck into the center of the cake comes out clean.
8. Place the cake on a cooling rack, and melt a few more tablespoons of butter on top if you wish.
9. Cut the pancake "cake" into 4 pieces and serve warm.

Per Serving

Calories: **502** | Fat: **43g** | Carbs: **13g** | Fiber: **5g** | Protein: **18g**

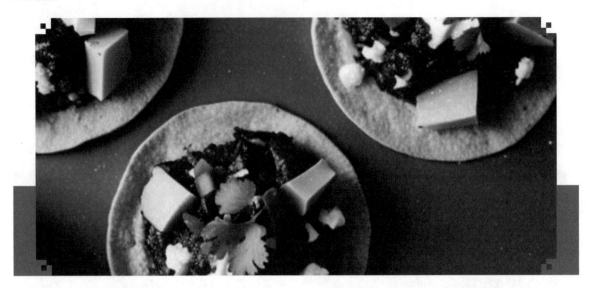

AVOCADO AND EGGS

Prep time: **10 minutes** | Cook time: **20 minutes** | Serves 4

- 2 avocados, peeled, halved lengthwise, and pitted
- 4 large eggs
- 1 (4-ounce) chicken breast, cooked and shredded
- ¼ cup Cheddar cheese
- Sea salt
- Freshly ground black pepper

1. Preheat the oven to 425°F.
2. Take a spoon and hollow out each side of the avocado halves until the hole is about twice the original size.
3. Place the avocado halves in an 8-by-8-inch baking dish, hollow-side up.
4. Crack an egg into each hollow and divide the shredded chicken between each avocado half. Sprinkle the cheese on top of each and season lightly with the salt and pepper.
5. Bake the avocados until the eggs are cooked through, about 15 to 20 minutes.
6. Serve immediately.

Per Serving

Calories: **324** | Fat: **25g** | Protein: **19g** | Carbs: **8g** | Fiber: **5g**

BREAKFAST TOSTADAS

Prep time: **10 minutes** | Cook time: **20 minutes** | Serves 4

- 1 peeled jicama
- 1 tablespoon coconut oil
- 4 cups cauliflower rice
- 2 teaspoons ground paprika
- 1 teaspoon ground coriander
- 2 teaspoons ground oregano
- 1 teaspoon ground cumin
- 2 avocados, sliced
- 1 cup fresh salsa, divided
- 1 cup sour cream
- ¼ cup chopped fresh cilantro

1. Using a mandoline or a chef's knife, slice the jicama into thin discs and set aside.
2. Warm the coconut oil in a large skillet over medium heat. Toss in the cauliflower rice, paprika, coriander, oregano, and cumin.
3. Cook, stirring often and allowing any excess water to cook off, for about 12 minutes.
4. Once the cauliflower starts to become tender, remove the skillet from the heat.
5. To make the tostadas, place the jicama slices on a platter.
6. On top of the disks, spoon the cauliflower, avocado, fresh salsa, sour cream, and cilantro.

Per Serving

Calories: **479** | Fat: **30g** | Carbs: **51g** | Fiber: **29g** | Protein: **13g**

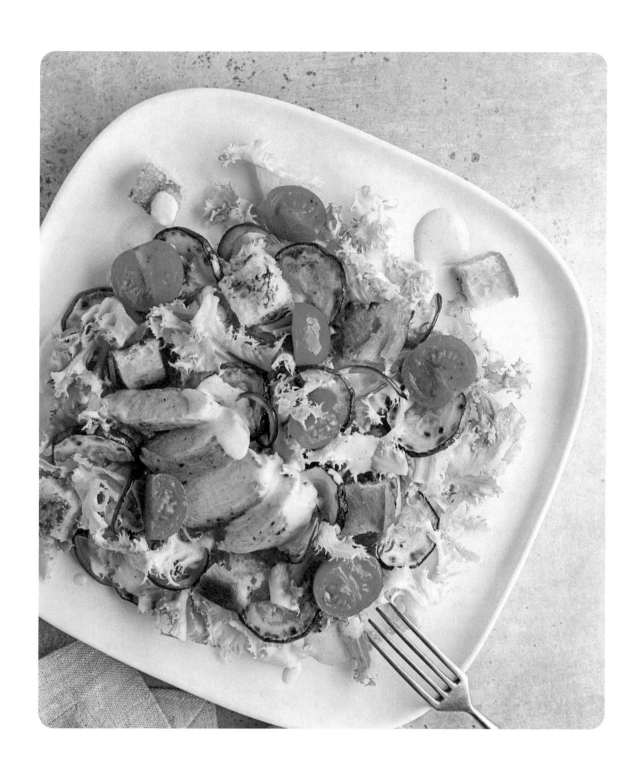

CHAPTER 4:
POULTRY

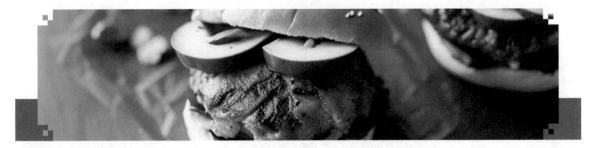

SPICY AVOCADO TURKEY BURGER

Prep time: **5 minutes** |Cook time: **10 minutes**| Serves 4

- 4 turkey burger patties
- 1 teaspoon salt
- 1 teaspoon freshly ground black pepper
- 4 slices pepper jack cheese
- 2 medium avocados, diced
- ½ medium onion, peeled and chopped
- 2 cloves garlic, pressed
- 3 tablespoons lime juice
- 3 tablespoons sriracha or other hot sauce

1. Season burgers with salt and pepper and cook on a preheated grill or grill pan over high heat 5–6 minutes per side or until fully cooked. Add cheese to burgers and cover during last minute of cook time to melt.
2. In a medium bowl, mash together avocado, onion, garlic, and lime juice, mixing until smooth.
3. Top each burger with avocado spread and sriracha and serve.

Per Serving

Calories: **348** | Fat: **25 g** | Protein: **25 g** | Fiber: **5 g** | Carbs: **8 g**

BALSAMIC CHICKEN AND VEGGIE SKEWERS

Prep time: **10 minutes** |Cook time: **50 minutes**| Serves 4

- 1½ cups quick brown rice
- 2 tablespoons balsamic vinegar
- 2 tablespoons olive oil
- ⅛ teaspoon Dijon mustard
- Sea salt
- Freshly ground black pepper
- 1 pound boneless, skinless chicken breast, cut
- into 1-inch pieces
- 1 medium zucchini, cut into 1-inch slices
- 1 yellow bell pepper, seeded and cut into 1-inch pieces
- 1 large white onion, peeled and cut into 16 wedges

1. Cook the rice according to the package instructions.
2. Soak 12 wooden skewers in warm water for 30 minutes.
3. In a large zip-top plastic bag, mix the balsamic vinegar, olive oil, mustard, salt, and pepper. Add the chicken and seal the bag, making sure to remove as much air as possible. Squish the chicken around in the bag to ensure that all the pieces are evenly coated. Refrigerate for at least 30 minutes.
4. Preheat the oven to 450°F. Line 2 baking sheets with aluminum foil.
5. Remove the chicken from the marinade and discard the marinade. Thread the chicken, zucchini, bell pepper, and onion on the skewers.
6. Place skewers on the prepared baking sheets and bake for 25 to 30 minutes, flipping the skewers after 15 minutes, or until cooked through.
7. Divide the rice between 4 plates and top with skewers of meat and vegetables.

Per Serving

Calories: **497**| Fat: **12g**| Carbs: **63g**| Fiber: **4g**| Protein: **32g**

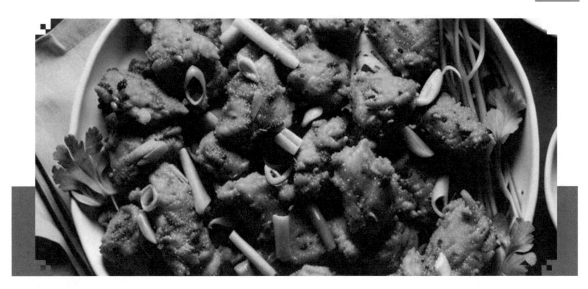

FRIED CHICKEN WITH COCONUT SAUCE

Prep time: 30 minutes | Cook time: 15 minutes | Serves 6

- 1 tbsp coconut oil
- 3 ½ pounds chicken breasts
- 1 cup chicken stock
- 1¼ cups leeks, chopped
- 1 tbsp lime juice
- ¼ cup coconut cream
- 2 tsp paprika
- 1 tsp red pepper flakes
- 2 tbsp green onions, chopped for garnishing
- Salt and ground black pepper, to taste

1. Set a pan over medium heat and warm oil, place in the chicken, cook each side for 2 minutes, set to a plate, and set aside. Set heat to medium, place the leeks to the pan and cook for 4 minutes.
2. Stir in the black pepper, stock, pepper flakes, salt, paprika, coconut cream, and lime juice. Take the chicken back to the pan, season with some more pepper and salt, and cook covered for 15 minutes.

Per Serving

Calories: **491** | Fat: **35g** | Carbs: **3.2g** | Protein: **58g** | Fiber: **4g**

TURKEY RISSOLES

Prep time: 10 minutes | Cook time: 25 minutes | Serves 4

- 1 pound ground turkey
- 1 scallion, white and green parts, finely chopped
- 1 teaspoon minced garlic
- Pinch sea salt
- Pinch freshly ground black pepper
- 1 cup ground almonds
- 2 tablespoons olive oil

1. Preheat the oven to 350°F. Line a baking sheet with aluminum foil and set aside.
2. In a medium bowl, mix together the turkey, scallion, garlic, salt, and pepper until well combined.
3. Shape the turkey mixture into 8 patties and flatten them out.
4. Place the ground almonds in a shallow bowl and dredge the turkey patties in the ground almonds to coat.
5. Place a large skillet over medium heat and add the olive oil.
6. Brown the turkey patties on both sides, about 10 minutes in total.
7. Transfer the patties to the baking sheet and bake them until cooked through, flipping them once, about 15 minutes in total.

Per Serving

Calories: **440** | Fat: **34g** | Protein: **27g** | Carbs: **7g** | Fiber: **4g**

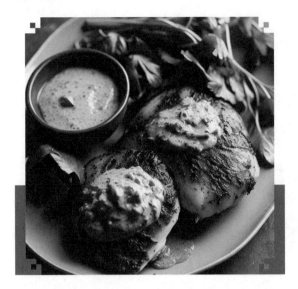

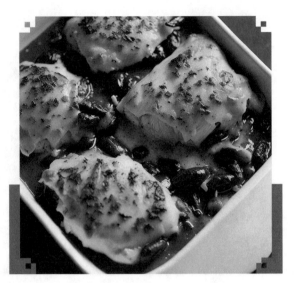

CILANTRO CHICKEN BREASTS

Prep time: 22 minutes | Cook time: 5 minutes | Serves 4

For The Sauce

- 1 avocado, pitted
- ½ cup mayonnaise
- Salt to taste

For The Chicken

- 1 tbsp ghee
- 2 chicken breasts
- Pink salt and black pepper to taste
- 1 cup chopped cilantro leaves
- ½ cup chicken broth

1. Spoon the avocado, mayonnaise, and salt into a small food processor and puree until a smooth sauce is derived. Pour sauce into a jar and refrigerate while you make the chicken.
2. Melt ghee in a large skillet, season chicken with salt and black pepper and fry for 4 minutes on each side to golden brown. Remove chicken to a plate.
3. Pour the broth in the same skillet and add the cilantro. Bring to simmer covered for 3 minutes and add the chicken. Cover and cook on low heat for 5 minutes until the liquid has reduced and chicken is fragrant. Dish chicken only into serving plates and spoon the mayoavocado sauce over.

Per Serving

Calories: 398 | Fat: 32g | Carbs: 4g | Protein: 24g| Fiber: 5.7g|

CHICKEN, EGGPLANT AND GRUYERE GRATIN

Prep time: 55 minutes | Cook time: 40 minutes | Serves 4

- 3 tbsp butter
- 1 eggplant, chopped
- 2 tbsp gruyere cheese, grated
- Salt and black pepper, to taste
- 2 garlic cloves, minced
- 6 chicken thighs

1. Set a pan over medium heat and warm 1 tablespoon butter, place in the chicken thighs, season with pepper and salt, cook each side for 3 minutes and lay them in a baking dish. In the same pan melt the rest of the butter and cook the garlic for 1 minute.
2. Stir in the eggplant, pepper, and salt, and cook for 10 minutes. Ladle this mixture over the chicken, spread with the cheese, set in the oven at 350ºF, and bake for 30 minutes. Turn on the oven's broiler, and broil everything for 2 minutes. Split among serving plates and enjoy.

Per Serving

Calories: 412 | Fat: 37g | Carbs: 5g | Protein: 34g | Fiber: 7.2 g

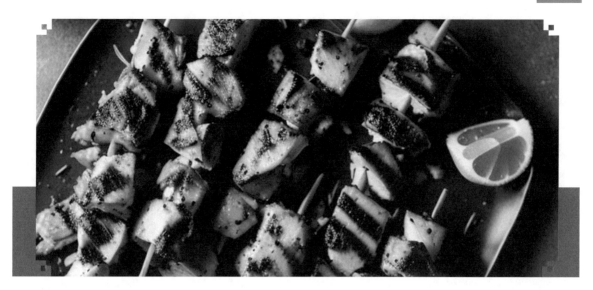

BACON & CHEESE CHICKEN

Prep time: 30 minutes | Cook time: 19 minutes | Serves 4

- 4 bacon strips
- 4 chicken breasts
- green onions, chopped
- ounces ranch dressing
- ounce coconut aminos
- tbsp coconut oil
- 4 oz Monterey Jack cheese, grated

1. Set a pan over high heat and warm the oil. Place in the chicken breasts, cook for 7 minutes, then flip to the other side; cook for an additional 7 minutes. Set another pan over medium heat, place in the bacon, cook until crispy, remove to paper towels, drain the grease, and crumble.
2. Add the chicken breast to a baking dish. Place the green onions, coconut aminos, cheese, and crumbled bacon on top, set in an oven, turn on the broiler, and cook for 5 minutes at high temperature. Split among serving plates and serve.

Per Serving

Calories: 423 | Fat: 21g | Carbs: 3.3g | Protein: 34g| Fiber: 4.7g

LEMON THREADED CHICKEN SKEWERS

Prep time: 2 hours 17 minutes | Cook time: 5 minutes | Serves 4

- 3 chicken breasts, cut into cubes
- 2 tbsp olive oil, divided
- ⅔ jar preserved lemon, flesh removed, drained
- 2 cloves garlic, minced
- ½ cup lemon juice
- Salt and black pepper to taste
- 1 tsp rosemary leaves to garnish
- 2 to 4 lemon wedges to garnish

1. First, thread the chicken onto skewers and set aside.
2. In a wide bowl, mix half of the oil, garlic, salt, pepper, and lemon juice, and add the chicken skewers, and lemon rind. Cover the bowl and let the chicken marinate for at least 2 hours in the refrigerator.
3. When the marinating time is almost over, preheat a grill to 350°F, and remove the chicken onto the grill. Cook for 6 minutes on each side.
4. Remove and serve warm garnished with rosemary leaves and lemons wedges.

Per Serving

Calories: 350 | Fat: 11g | Carbs: 3.5g | Protein: 34g |Fiber: 5.4 g

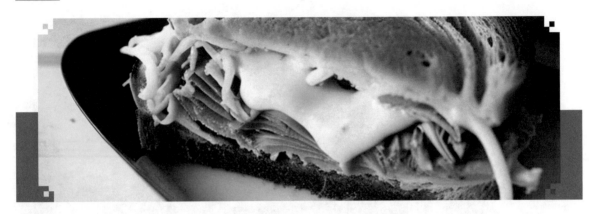

TURKEY REUBEN SANDWICHES

Prep time: **5 minutes** |Cook time: **15 minutes**| Serves **4**

- 2 tablespoons olive oil
- 6 ounces sliced turkey
- 4 slices reduced-fat Swiss cheese
- 1 cup sauerkraut, drained
- ½ cup fat-free Thousand Island dressing
- 8 slices rye bread

1. Heat oil in a nonstick skillet over medium heat.
2. While pan heats, evenly divide turkey, cheese, sauerkraut, and dressing between the slices of rye bread, stacking two with toppings, then topping with the remaining two slices.
3. Cook sandwich in skillet 3 minutes per side, until bread is toasted and warm, then serve.

Per Serving

Calories: **403** | Fat: **15 g** | Protein: **23 g** |Fiber: **6 g** | Carbs: **43 g**

CHICKEN WITH MANGO SALSA

Prep time: **10 minutes** |Cook time: **25 minutes**| Serves **4**

- 1 tablespoon olive oil
- 4 (4-ounce) boneless, skinless chicken breasts
- ½ teaspoon sea salt
- ¼ teaspoon freshly ground black pepper
- 1 avocado, pitted, peeled, and diced
- 1 cup diced fresh or frozen mango
- 1 garlic clove, minced
- ¼ cup minced red onion
- ¼ cup chopped fresh cilantro
- 2 tablespoons lime juice
- 1 teaspoon olive oil
- 8 cups mixed greens

1. Preheat the oven to 400°F. Line a baking sheet with aluminum foil.
2. Using a basting brush, spread the olive oil over the chicken and season with the salt and pepper. Arrange the chicken on the prepared baking sheet and bake for 20 to 25 minutes, or until cooked through.
3. While the chicken bakes, in a large bowl, mix the avocado, mango, garlic, red onion, and cilantro. Add the lime juice and oil and stir until combined. Cover with plastic wrap and refrigerate until ready to serve.
4. Place a chicken breast on each of 4 plates. Divide the mixed greens between the plates and top with mango salsa.

Per Serving

Calories: **313**| Fat: **16g**| Carbs: **16g**| Fiber: **6g**| Protein: **29g**

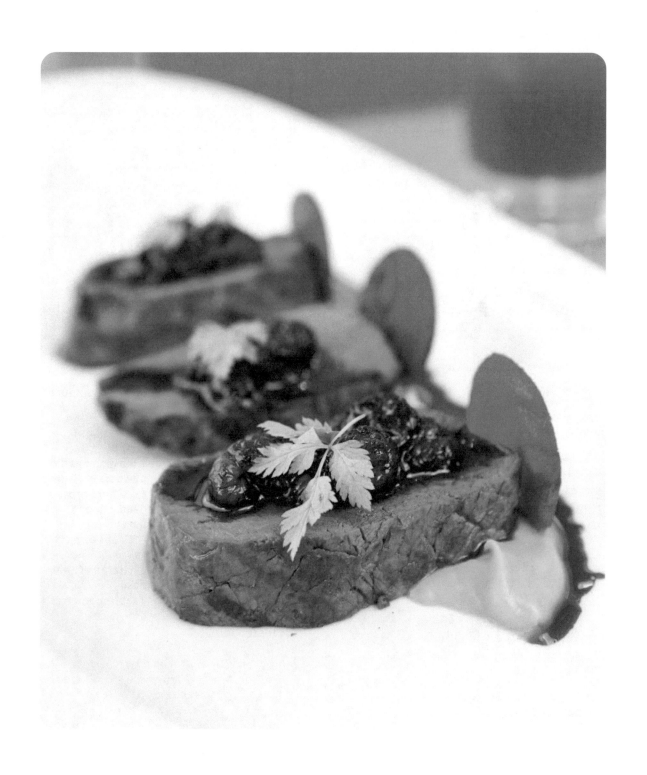

CHAPTER 5: RED MEAT AND PORK

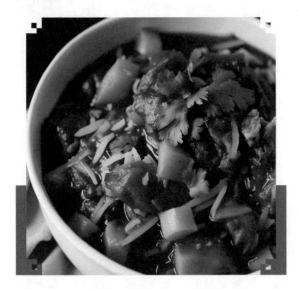

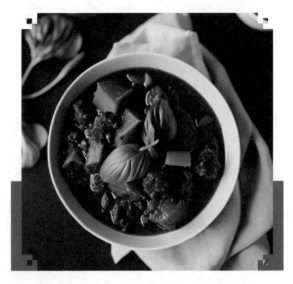

PORK-AND-SAUERKRAUT CASSEROLE

Prep time: 15 minutes | Cook time: 9 to 10 hours | Serves 6

- 3 tablespoons extra-virgin olive oil, divided
- 2 tablespoons butter
- 2 pounds pork shoulder roast
- 1 (28-ounce) jar sauerkraut, drained
- 1 cup chicken broth
- ½ sweet onion, thinly sliced
- ¼ cup granulated erythritol

1. Lightly grease the insert of the slow cooker with 1 tablespoon of the olive oil.
2. In a large skillet over medium-high heat, heat the remaining 2 tablespoons of the olive oil and the butter. Add the pork to the skillet and brown on all sides for about 10 minutes.
3. Transfer to the insert and add the sauerkraut, broth, onion, and erythritol.
4. Cover and cook on low for 9 to 10 hours.
5. Serve warm.

Per Serving

Calories: 516 | Fat: 42g | Protein: 28g | Carbs: 7g | Fiber: 4g

THAI GROUND BEEF CURRY

Prep time: 10 minutes | Cook time: 35 minutes | Serves 6

- 2 teaspoons tallow, at room temperature
- 1 ½ pounds ground chuck
- 1 shallot, chopped
- 1 teaspoon ginger-garlic paste
- 1 teaspoon red curry paste
- ½ teaspoon turmeric
- ½ teaspoon cumin
- ½ teaspoon salt
- 1/3 teaspoon pepper
- 1 teaspoon garlic powder
- 1 medium broccoli head, chopped into florets
- 1 ½ cups tomato sauce
- 1 handful of Thai basil
- 1 tablespoon fresh lime juice

1. In a deep saucepan, melt the tallow for a few minutes. Once hot, brown the ground meat for 5 to 6 minutes, crumbling with a fork.
2. Add the remaining ingredients to the saucepan and stir to combine. Reduce the heat to simmer; let it simmer, partially covered, for 25 minutes or until thoroughly cooked.
3. Ladle into individual bowls and serve warm. Bon appétit!

Per Serving

Calories: 216 | Fat: 10.6g | Carbs: 5.2g | Protein: 24.8g | Fiber: 2.5g

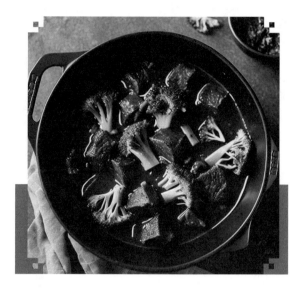
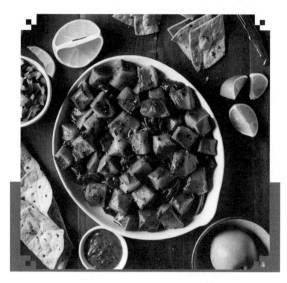

BEEF AND BROCCOLI ROAST

Prep time: 10 minutes | Cook time: 4 hours 30 minutes | Serves 2

- 1 pound beef chuck roast
- Pink Himalayan salt
- Freshly ground black pepper
- ½ cup beef broth, plus more if needed
- ¼ cup soy sauce (or coconut aminos)
- 1 teaspoon toasted sesame oil
- 1 (16-ounce) bag frozen broccoli

1. with the crock insert in place, preheat the slow cooker to low.
2. On a cutting board, season the chuck roast with pink Himalayan salt and pepper, and slice the roast thin. Put the sliced beef in the slow cooker.
3. In a small bowl, mix together the beef broth, soy sauce, and sesame oil. Pour over the beef.
4. Cover and cook on low for 4 hours.
5. Add the frozen broccoli, and cook for 30 minutes more. If you need more liquid, add additional beef broth.
6. Serve hot.

Per Serving

Calories: **806** | Fat: **49g** | Carbs: **18g** Fiber: **6g** | Protein: **74g**

CRISPY MEXICAN PORK CARNITAS

Prep time: 5 minutes | Cook time: 45 minutes |Serves 4

- 2 pounds pork butt, cut into 2-inch cubes
- ½ cup dry red wine
- ½ cup tomato sauce
- ½ cup chicken stock
- 2 tablespoons tomato ketchup
- 2 tablespoons Dijon mustard
- 1 teaspoon celery seeds
- 1 teaspoon fennel seeds
- 4 tablespoons scallions, chopped
- 2 garlic cloves, minced

1. Brush a stockpot or Dutch oven with nonstick cooking spray. Preheat your pot over mediumhigh heat and sear the pork butt until brown and cooked through.
2. After your pork is browned, add the remaining ingredients to the stockpot. Stir to combine well.
3. Transfer the mixture to a baking dish. Cover with foil and bake in the preheated oven at 350 degrees F for about 35 minutes.
4. Switch your oven to broil. Now, broil the meat for approximately 7 minutes, until the top is slightly crisp. Serve immediately and enjoy!

Per Serving

Calories: **477** | Fat: **16.2g** | Carbs: **5.7g** | Protein: **67.7g** | Fiber: **2.2g**

39

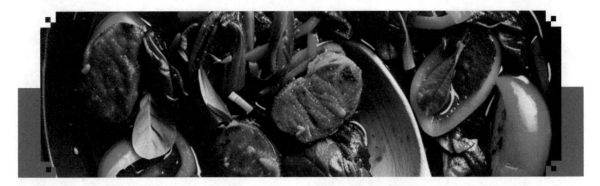

STICKY BARBECUED RIBS

Prep time: 10 minutes | Cook time: 1 hour 45 minutes |Serves 4

- 1 tablespoon olive oil
- 1 pound beef ribs
- 1 leek, sliced
- ½ cup red wine
- 1 cup vegetable broth
- 1 teaspoon cumin powder
- 1 teaspoon ginger powder
- Kosher salt and cayenne pepper, to taste
- 2 teaspoons liquid smoke
- 2 teaspoons granulated garlic
- ½ teaspoon stevia powder
- 2 teaspoons American-style mustard
- 2 tablespoons sesame seeds, toasted
- 4 tablespoons fresh chives, chopped

1. Heat the olive oil in a pan over a moderate flame. Now, sear the beef ribs for 3 to 4 minutes on each side; stir in the leek and cook an additional 3 minutes.
2. Add a splash of wine to deglaze the pan. Now, add in the remaining wine, broth, cumin powder, ginger powder, salt, and pepper.
3. Decrease the temperature to medium-low, cover, and let it cook for 40 minutes. Now, line a baking dish with foil. Place the ribs along with the cooking liquid in the baking dish.
4. Add in the liquid smoke, garlic, stevia, and American-style mustard. Bake in the preheated oven at 300 degrees F for 1 hour; make sure to turn the ribs periodically to ensure they are coated with the glaze.
5. Top with sesame seeds and chives. Bon appétit!

Per Serving

Calories: **481** | Fat: **41g** | Carbs: **5.9g** | Protein: **19.9g** | Fiber: **1.3g**

PORK SAUSAGE STUFFED TOMATOES WITH CHEESE

Prep time: 5 minutes | Cook time: 50 minutes |Serves 4

- 4 ounces pork sausage, sliced
- 1 onion, chopped
- 1 garlic clove, minced
- Sea salt and ground black pepper, to season
- ½ teaspoon mustard seeds
- ½ teaspoon celery seeds
- 4 tomatoes
- 2 ounces cream cheese
- 4 ounces Colby cheese, shredded

1. In a nonstick skillet over a moderate flame, brown the pork sausage for 5 minutes, crumbling it with a fork.
2. Now, fold in the onion and garlic and cook for a further 3 minutes. Stir in the salt, black pepper, mustard seeds, and celery seeds.
3. Using a sharp knife, slice a thin piece off the top of each tomato. Scoop out the pulp, leaving a ½-inch shell.
4. Spoon the filling into the tomatoes. Place the stuffed tomatoes in a baking dish and cover them with aluminum foil. Bake in the preheated oven at 360 degrees F for about 35 minutes.
5. Spoon the cream cheese and Colby cheese on top of each tomato. Bake an additional 6 minutes. Bon appétit!

Per Serving

Calories: **300** | Fat: **21.9g** | Carbs: **9g** | Protein: **14.3g** | Fiber: **2g**

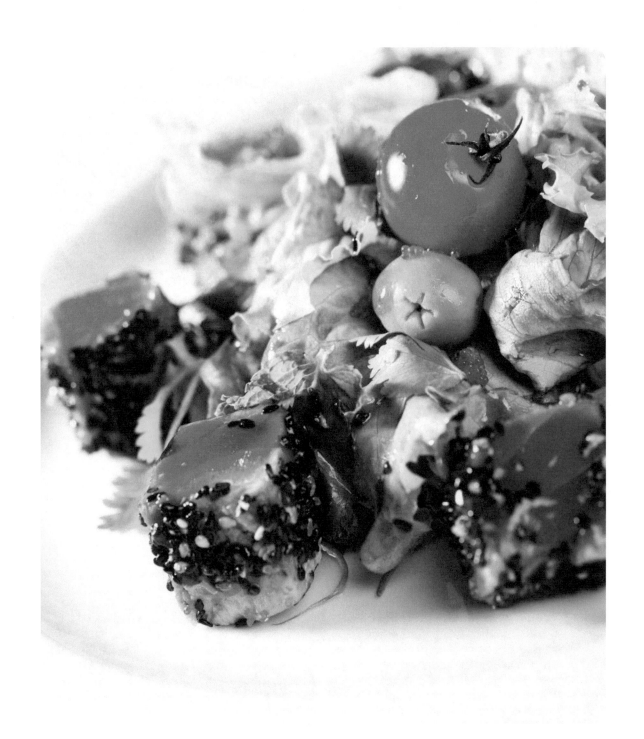

CHAPTER 6: FISH AND SEAFOOD

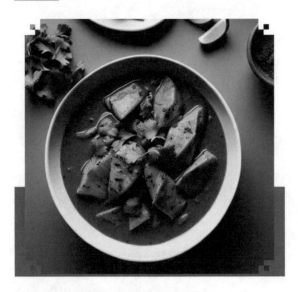

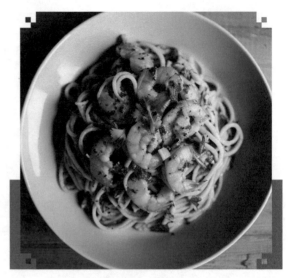

FISH CURRY MASALA

Prep time: **5 minutes** | **Cook time: 25 minutes** |**Serves 6**

- 2 tablespoons sesame oil
- 1 shallot, chopped
- 2 bell peppers, deveined and sliced
- 1 teaspoon coriander, ground
- 1 teaspoon cumin, ground
- 4 tablespoons red curry paste
- 1 teaspoon ginger-garlic paste
- 1 ½ pounds white fish fillets, skinless, boneless
- ½ cup tomato sauce
- ½ cup haddi ka shorba (Indian bone broth)
- 1 cup coconut milk
- ½ teaspoon red chili powder
- Kosher salt and ground black pepper, to taste

1. Heat the sesame oil in a saucepan over moderate heat; then, sauté the shallot and peppers until they have softened or about 4 minutes.
2. Now, stir in the coriander, cumin, red curry paste, and ginger-garlic paste; continue to sauté an additional 4 minutes, stirring frequently.
3. After that, fold in the fish and tomato sauce; pour in the haddi ka shorba and coconut milk. Season with red chili powder, salt, and black pepper.
4. Turn the heat to simmer and let it cook for 5 minutes longer or until everything is cooked through. Enjoy!

Per Serving

Calories: 349 | Fat: 24.9g | Carbs: 6.2g | Protein: 22.7g | Fiber: 2.5g

SHRIMP SCAMPI WITH WHOLE WHEAT PASTA

Prep time: **15 minutes** | **Cook time: 20 minutes** | **Serves 4**

- 1 pound large shrimp, peeled and deveined
- ½ pound whole wheat pasta
- 2 tablespoons olive oil
- 3 cloves garlic, minced
- ½ cup white wine
- ¼ cup fresh lemon juice
- ¼ cup chopped parsley
- Salt and pepper to taste

1. Cook the pasta according to package instructions.
2. Heat olive oil in a large skillet over medium-high heat. Add shrimp and cook for 2-3 minutes per side, or until pink and cooked through. Remove shrimp from skillet and set aside.
3. Add garlic to the skillet and cook for 1 minute, or until fragrant. Deglaze the skillet with white wine and lemon juice. Bring to a simmer and cook for 2-3 minutes, or until sauce has thickened.
4. Toss cooked pasta with the shrimp and sauce. Garnish with parsley and serve immediately.

Per Serving

Calories: 350 | Fat: 15g | Carbs: 40g | Protein: 30g | Fiber: 5g

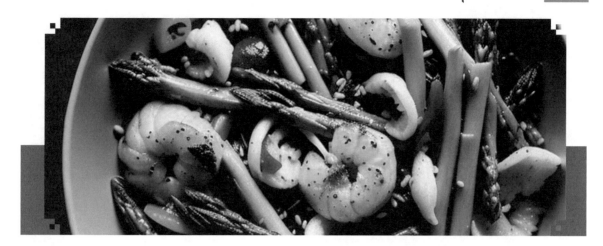

FISH TACO BOWL

Prep time: 10 minutes | Cook time: 15 minutes | Serves 2

- 2 (5-ounce) tilapia fillets
- 1 tablespoon olive oil
- 4 teaspoons Tajín seasoning salt, divided
- 2 cups presliced coleslaw cabbage mix
- 1 tablespoon Spicy Red Pepper Miso Mayo, plus more for serving
- 1 avocado, mashed
- Pink Himalayan salt
- Freshly ground black pepper

1. Preheat the oven to 425°F. Line a baking sheet with aluminum foil or a silicone baking mat.
2. Rub the tilapia with the olive oil, and then coat it with 2 teaspoons of Tajín seasoning salt. Place the fish in the prepared pan.
3. Bake for 15 minutes, or until the fish is opaque when you pierce it with a fork. Put the fish on a cooling rack and let it sit for 4 minutes.
4. Meanwhile, in a medium bowl, gently mix to combine the coleslaw and the mayo sauce. You don't want the cabbage super wet, just enough to dress it. Add the mashed avocado and the remaining 2 teaspoons of Tajín seasoning salt to the coleslaw, and season with pink Himalayan salt and pepper. Divide the salad between two bowls.
5. Use two forks to shred the fish into small pieces, and add it to the bowls.
6. Top the fish with a drizzle of mayo sauce and serve.

Per Serving

Calories: **315** | Fat: **24g** | Carbs: **12g** | Fiber: **7g** | Protein: **16g**

ASIAN SEAFOOD STIR-FRY

Prep time: 10 minutes | Cook time:15 minutes |Serves 4

- 4 teaspoons sesame oil
- ½ cup yellow onion, sliced
- 1 cup asparagus spears, sliced
- ½ cup celery, chopped
- ½ cup enoki mushrooms
- 1 pound bay scallops
- 1 tablespoon fresh parsley, chopped
- Kosher salt and ground black pepper, to taste
- ½ teaspoon red pepper flakes, crushed
- 1 tablespoon coconut aminos
- 2 tablespoons rice wine
- ½ cup dry roasted peanuts, roughly chopped

1. Heat 1 teaspoon of the sesame oil in a wok over a medium-high flame. Now, fry the onion until crisp-tender and translucent; reserve.
2. Heat another teaspoon of the sesame oil and fry the asparagus and celery for about 3 minutes until crisp-tender; reserve.
3. Then, heat another teaspoon of the sesame oil and cook the mushrooms for 2 minutes more or until they start to soften; reserve.
4. Lastly, heat the remaining teaspoon of sesame oil and cook the bay scallops just until they are opaque.
5. Return all reserved vegetables to the wok. Add in the remaining ingredients and toss to combine. Serve warm and enjoy!

Per Serving

Calories: **236** | Fat: **12.5g** | Carbs: **5.9g** | Protein: **27g** | Fiber: **2.4g**

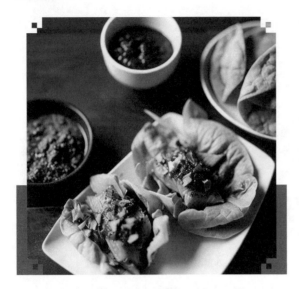

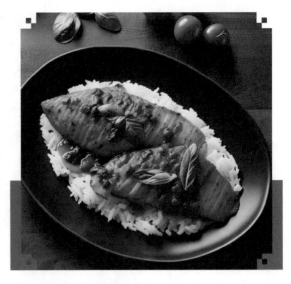

SALMON LETTUCE TACOS WITH GUAJILLO SAUCE

Prep time: 5 minutes | Cook time: 20 minutes |Serves 5

- 2 pounds salmon
- Flaky salt and ground black pepper, to taste
- 10 lettuce leaves
- 2 bell peppers, chopped
- 1 cucumber, chopped
- 1 avocado, pitted and peeled
- 1 tomato, halved
- 2 tablespoons extra-virgin olive oil
- 1 tablespoon lemon juice
- 4 tablespoons green onions
- 1 teaspoon garlic
- 1 guajillo chili pepper

1. Season your salmon with salt and black pepper. Brush the salmon on all sides with nonstick cooking oil.
2. Grill over medium heat for 13 minutes until golden and opaque in the middle. Flake the fish with two forks.
3. Divide the fish among the lettuce leaves; add the bell peppers and cucumber.
4. Pulse the remaining ingredients in your blender 8 to 10 times or until smooth with several small chunks of tomatoes and scallions.
5. Top each lettuce taco with the guajillo sauce and serve.

Per Serving

Calories: 342 | Fat: 16.5g | Carbs: 6.8g | Protein: 40g | Fiber: 40g

TILAPIA WITH OLIVES & TOMATO SAUCE

Prep time: 30 minutes | Cook time: 38 minutes | Serves 4

- 4 tilapia fillets
- 2 garlic cloves, minced
- 1 tsp oregano
- 14 unces diced tomatoes
- 1 tbsp olive oil
- ½ red onion, chopped
- 1 tbsp parsley
- ¼ cup kalamata olives

1. Heat olive oil in a skillet over medium heat and cook the onion for 3 minutes. Add garlic and oregano and cook for 30 seconds. Stir in tomatoes and bring the mixture to a boil.
2. Reduce the heat and simmer for 5 minutes. Add olives and tilapia, and cook for about 8 minutes. Serve the tilapia with tomato sauce.

Per Serving

Calories: 282 | Fat: 15g | Carbs: 6g | Protein: 23g| Fiber:3.5g

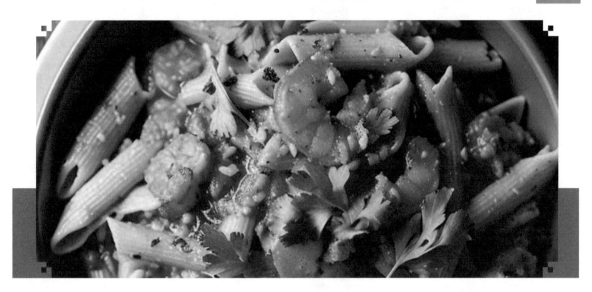

GRILLED TUNA STEAKS WITH ROASTED ASPARAGUS

Prep time: 15 minutes | Cook time: **15 minutes** | Serves 2

- 2 tuna steaks
- 1 bunch asparagus
- 1 tablespoon olive oil
- Salt and pepper to taste

1. Preheat oven to 400°F. Toss asparagus in olive oil, salt, and pepper. Roast for 10-12 minutes, or until tender-crisp.
2. Season tuna steaks with salt and pepper. Grill for 3-4 minutes per side, or until cooked to your desired doneness.
3. Serve grilled tuna steaks with roasted asparagus.

Per Serving

Calories: 350 | Fat: **20g** | Carbs: **10g** | Protein: **40g** | Fiber: **3g**

MEDITERRANEAN SHRIMP PENNE

Prep time: 5 minutes | Cook time: **20 minutes** | Serves 4

- 1 (16-ounce) package whole-grain penne
- 2 tablespoons olive oil
- ¼ cup chopped red onion
- 1 tablespoon chopped garlic
- ¼ cup white wine
- 2 (12-ounce) cans diced tomatoes
- 1 pound shrimp, peeled and deveined
- 1 cup grated Parmesan cheese

1. Cook pasta according to package directions and set aside.
2. Heat oil in a medium nonstick skillet over medium-high heat. Add onion and garlic, cooking about 5 minutes until onion becomes tender.
3. Add wine and tomatoes and cook 10 more minutes, stirring frequently.
4. Add shrimp to sauce and cook an additional 5 minutes. Toss shrimp with pasta and serve with Parmesan sprinkled on top.

Per Serving

Calories: 658 | Fat: **18 g** | Protein: **37 g** | Fiber: **12 g** | Carbs: **90 g**

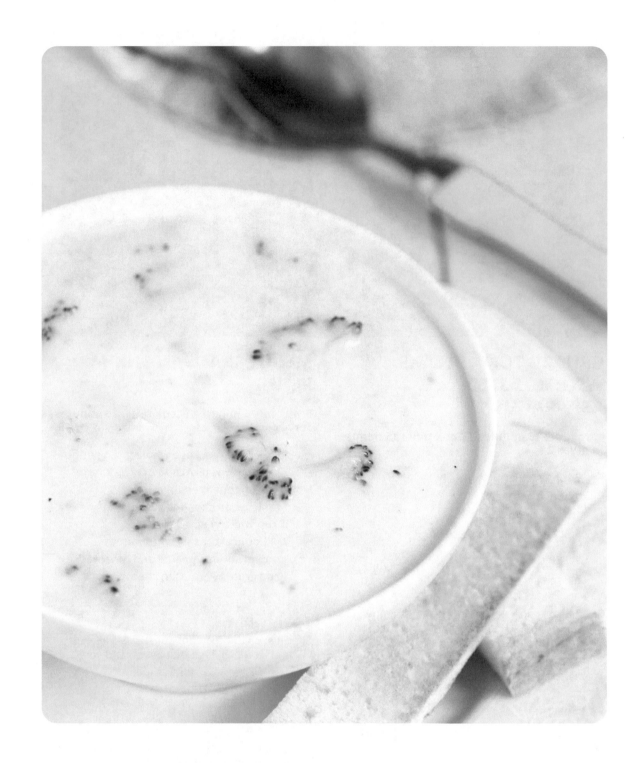

CHAPTER 7:
VEGETARIAN SIDES
AND SOUPS

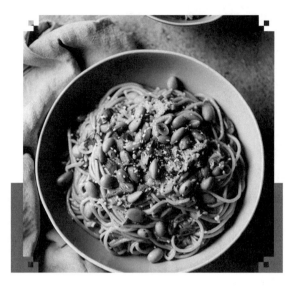

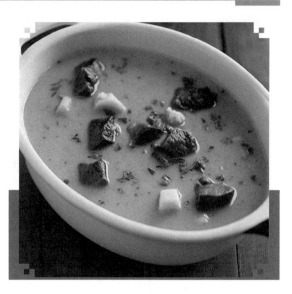

CHEESY EDAMAME SPAGHETTI

Prep time: 5 minutes | Cook time: 10 minutes | Serves 4

- 4 ounces brown rice spaghetti
- 1 cup unsalted roasted cashews
- ⅓ cup grated parmesan cheese
- 1 teaspoon garlic powder
- ½ teaspoon salt
- 3 cups frozen edamame, thawed
- 2 cups finely chopped fresh parsley
- 2 teaspoons extra-virgin olive oil
- ½ teaspoon ground black pepper

1. Fill a large pot with water and bring to a boil over high heat. Add pasta and cook for 10 minutes. Drain and transfer to a large bowl.
2. Add cashews, cheese, garlic powder, and salt to a food processor. Pulse until a coarse texture is achieved. Set aside.
3. Toss pasta with edamame, parsley, oil, and pepper. Top with cashew mixture, toss to combine, and serve.

Per Serving

Calories: 568 | Fat: 30g | Carbs: 49g | Fiber: 17g | Protein: 25g

SLOW COOKER LAMB & CAULIFLOWER SOUP

Prep time: 10 minutes | Cook time: 4 hours | Serves 6

- 1 pound ground lamb
- 5 cups beef broth
- 1 cauliflower head, cut into florets
- 1 cup heavy cream
- 1 yellow onion, chopped
- 2 cloves garlic, chopped
- 1 tablespoon freshly chopped thyme
- ½ teaspoon cracked black pepper
- ½ teaspoon salt

1. Add the ground lamb and cauliflower to the base of a stockpot.
2. Add in the remaining ingredients minus the heavy cream, and cook on high for 4 hours.
3. Warm the heavy cream before adding to the soup. Use an immersion blender to blend the soup until creamy.

Per Serving

Calories: 263 | Carbs: 6g | Fiber: 2g | Fat: 14g | Protein: 27g

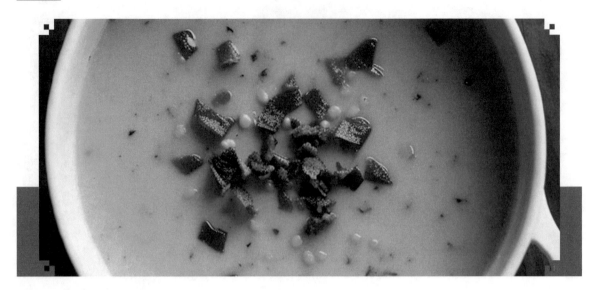

CILANTRO LIME RICE

Prep time: **5 minutes** | Cook time: **5 minutes** | Serves **4**

- 1 (10-ounce) bag riced cauliflower (thawed or fresh)
- 3 tablespoons water
- 1 medium lime, juiced and zested
- ½ cup chopped cilantro

1. Combine riced cauliflower and water in a large microwave-safe bowl and microwave 3–5 minutes or until cauliflower is soft.
2. Remove and add lime juice, zest, and cilantro to bowl. Mix well before serving.

Per Serving

Calories: 176 | Fat: 2 g | Protein: 14 g | Fiber: 17 g | Carbs: 35 g

CORN AND BACON CHOWDER

Prep time: **5 minutes** | Cook time: **5 minutes** | Serves **4**

- ½ cup chopped celery
- ½ cup chopped onion
- 2 (16-ounce) packages frozen corn, thawed and divided
- 2 cups skim milk, divided
- ½ teaspoon salt
- ¼ teaspoon freshly ground black pepper
- ¾ cup fat-free shredded Cheddar cheese
- 2 slices bacon, cooked and crumbled

1. Sauté celery, onion, and 1 package corn in a stockpot over medium heat 5 minutes or until tender.
2. In a blender, blend the remaining package corn and 1 cup skim milk until smooth.
3. Add blended corn and milk mixture to pan with vegetables. Add remaining milk, salt, pepper, and cheese.
4. Cook, stirring constantly, until cheese melts. Serve topped with crumbled bacon bits.

Per Serving

Calories: 347 | Fat: 9 g | Protein: 20 g | Fiber: 7 g | Carbs: 56 g

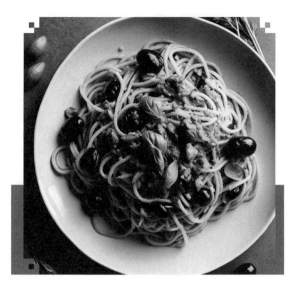

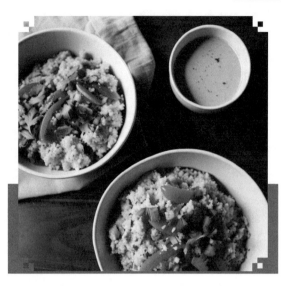

PASTA WITH PESTO AND OLIVE SAUCE

Prep time: 5 minutes | **Cook time: 5 minutes** | **Serves 4**

- 1 (16-ounce) package spaghetti
- ½ cup reserved pasta water
- 2 cloves garlic
- ¼ cup olive oil
- ¼ cup green olives
- ¼cup fresh parsley
- ¼ cup fresh basil
- ¼ cup black olives
- ½ teaspoon salt

1. Cook the spaghetti al dente according to package directions and drain, reserving ½ cup pasta water.
2. To make the pesto, combine garlic, olive oil, green olives, parsley, and basil in a blender and blend thoroughly.
3. Transfer pesto to a large saucepan and heat 2 minutes over medium heat until warm.
4. Add spaghetti, black olives, salt, and reserved water to the saucepan and continue cooking until water is absorbed and spaghetti is heated. Serve immediately.

Per Serving

Calories: 320 | Fat: 17 g | Protein: 7 g | Fiber: 3 g | Carbs: 36 g

VEGETABLE COUSCOUS WITH PEANUT SAUCE

Prep time: 5 minutes | **Cook time: 10 minutes** | **Serves 2**

- 1 cup water
- 1 tablespoon salted butter or ghee
- 1 cup couscous
- ½ teaspoon salt
- 2 cups frozen mixed vegetables (peas, corn, carrots, and green beans), thawed
- 1 tablespoon Easy Peanut Sauce

1. In a medium saucepan, bring water and butter to a boil over high heat. Remove pan from the heat and stir in couscous and salt. Cover and set aside for 15 minutes.
2. Add vegetables to couscous in the pan and stir to combine.
3. Drizzle with Easy Peanut Sauce and serve immediately.

Per Serving

Calories: 471 | Fat: 10g | Carbs: 79g | Fiber: 6g | Protein: 13g

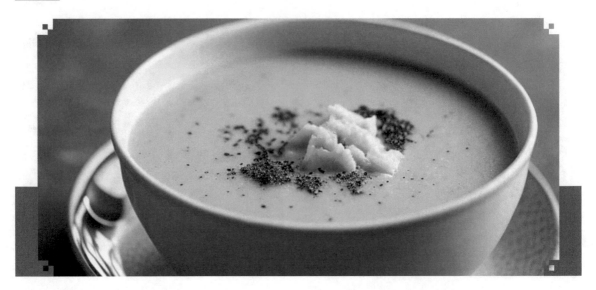

EGGPLANT PIZZAS

Prep time: 5 minutes | **Cook time:** 10 minutes | **Serves 4**

- 1 large eggplant, cut into ½" slices
- ¼ cup extra-virgin olive oil
- ¼ teaspoon salt
- ¼ teaspoon ground black pepper
- ¾ cup tomato sauce
- ½ teaspoon italian seasoning
- 4 ounces part-skim mozzarella cheese, thinly sliced
- 2 tablespoons minced fresh basil

1. Preheat broiler and line a baking sheet with parchment paper.
2. Brush each side of eggplant slices with oil and season with salt and pepper.
3. Heat a large nonstick skillet over medium heat. Cook eggplant slices in batches until tender and lightly browned, about 3–5 minutes per side.
4. Transfer eggplant slices to the prepared baking sheet and top each with tomato sauce, Italian seasoning, and cheese.
5. Broil for 3–5 minutes until cheese is melted and lightly browned.
6. Top with basil and serve.

Per Serving

Calories: 248 | **Fat: 17g** | **Carbs: 12g** | **Fiber: 5g** | **Protein: 11g**

GARLIC CHEDDAR CAULIFLOWER SOUP

Prep time: 5 minutes | **Cook time:** 10 minutes | **Serves 2**

- 2 tablespoons olive oil
- 1 small yellow onion, peeled and chopped
- 2 cloves garlic, peeled and minced
- 1 medium head cauliflower, cored, outer leaves removed, and chopped
- 4 cups low-sodium chicken broth
- ½ cup shredded sharp cheddar cheese
- ¼ cup grated parmesan cheese

1. Heat oil in a large saucepan over medium heat. Sauté onion and garlic 5 minutes.
2. Add cauliflower and broth. Increase heat to high and bring to a boil.
3. Reduce heat to medium-low and simmer 20 minutes until cauliflower is soft.
4. Remove from heat, then transfer soup to a blender and process until smooth (or use a handheld blender).
5. Return soup to pot, stir in Cheddar and Parmesan, and heat, stirring constantly, over medium heat 5 minutes until cheeses melt. Serve hot.

Per Serving

Calories: 351 | **Fat: 23g** | **Carbs: 18g** | **Fiber: 7g** | **Protein: 18g**

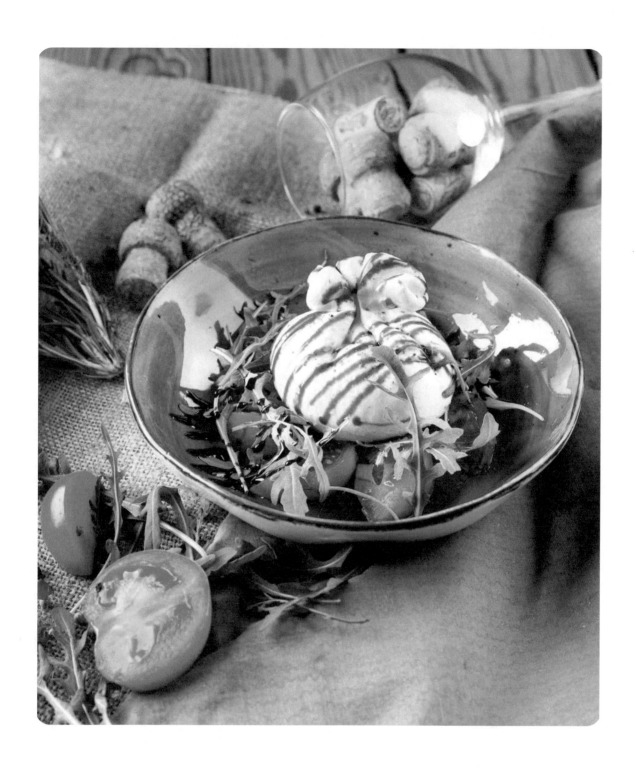

CHAPTER 8:
SALADS

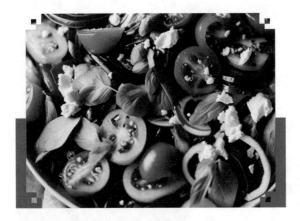

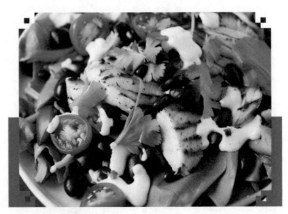

MEDITERRANEAN-STYLE ZUCCHINI SALAD

Prep time: 10 minutes | Cook time: 15 minutes | Serves 5

- 1 ½ pounds zucchini, sliced
- 4 tablespoons extra-virgin olive oil, divided
- Sea salt and ground black pepper, to taste
- ½ teaspoon cayenne pepper
- ½ teaspoon dried dill weed
- ½ teaspoon dried basil
- 1 red onion, sliced
- 1 garlic clove, pressed
- 2 tomatoes, sliced
- 1 teaspoon Dijon mustard
- 1 tablespoon balsamic vinegar
- 1 tablespoon fresh lime juice
- 4 ounces goat cheese, crumbled

1. Toss the zucchini with 2 tablespoons of olive oil and spices. Arrange them on a rimmed baking sheet.
2. Roast in the preheated oven at 425 degrees F until tender about 9 minutes. Toss roasted zucchini with red onion, garlic, and tomatoes.
3. Add the remaining tablespoons of olive oil, mustard, vinegar, and lime juice. Toss to combine and top with goat cheese. Enjoy!

Per Serving

Calories: 186 | Fat: 13.5g | Carbs: 6.6g | Protein: 11.2g | Fiber: 2.2g

BLACK BEAN AND CORN CHICKEN SALAD

Prep time: 10 minutes | Cook time: 15 minutes | Serves 2

- 2 teaspoons lime juice
- 2½ teaspoons olive oil, divided
- ½ teaspoon garlic powder
- 10 ounces boneless, skinless chicken breasts, cut into bite-size pieces
- Sea salt
- Freshly ground black pepper
- ½ cup frozen corn kernels
- 1 cup canned black beans, drained and rinsed
- 4 cups mixed greens
- ½ cup baby tomatoes, halved
- 2 scallions, green parts only, thinly sliced
- 1 cup fat-free sour cream

1. In a small bowl, mix the lime juice, ½ teaspoon of olive oil, and garlic powder. Set aside.
2. In a large nonstick skillet, heat the remaining 2 teaspoons of olive oil over medium-high heat. Add the chicken and cook, stirring occasionally, until golden brown and cooked through, 8 to 11 minutes. Season with salt and pepper to taste. Set aside.
3. While the chicken is cooking, in a small saucepan, cook the frozen corn according to the package instructions. Drain the corn.
4. In a medium bowl, mix the corn, black beans, greens, tomatoes, and scallions. Drizzle with the lime juice dressing and mix again. Divide the mixture equally between 2 bowls and top with the chicken and dollops of sour cream. Season with salt and pepper to taste, and serve immediately.

Per Serving

Calories: 424 | Fat: 10g | Carbs: 41g | Fiber: 9g | Protein: 43g

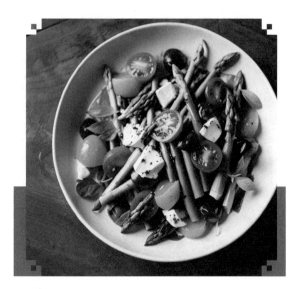

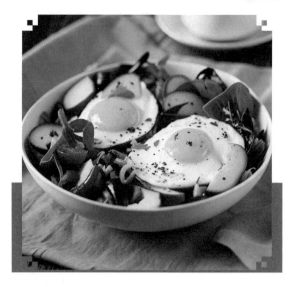

CAPRESE ASPARAGUS SALAD

Prep time: 5 minutes | Cook time: 20 minutes | Serves 4

- 1 teaspoon fresh lime juice
- 1 tablespoon hot Hungarian paprika infused oil
- ½ teaspoon kosher salt
- ¼ teaspoon red pepper flakes
- ½ pound asparagus spears, trimmed
- 1 cup grape tomatoes, halved
- 2 tablespoon red wine vinegar
- 1 garlic clove, pressed 1-2 drops liquid stevia
- 1 tablespoon fresh basil
- 1 tablespoon fresh chives
- ½ cup mozzarella, grated

1. Heat your grill to the hottest setting. Toss your asparagus with the lime juice, hot Hungarian paprika infused oil, salt, and red pepper flakes.
2. Place the asparagus spears on the hot grill. Grill until one side chars; then, grill your asparagus on the other side.
3. Cut the asparagus spears into bite-sized pieces and transfer to a salad bowl. Add the grape tomatoes, red wine, garlic, stevia, basil, and chives; toss to combine well.
4. Top with freshly grated mozzarella cheese and serve immediately.

Per Serving

Calories: **187** | Fat: **13.3g** | Carbs: **7.4g** | Protein: **9.5g** | Fiber: **3.4g**

PAN-FRIED EGG SALAD

Prep time: 5 minutes | Cook time:15 minutes | Serves 4

- 2 tablespoons canola oil
- 4 eggs
- 4 cups lettuce, broken into pieces
- 1 Lebanese cucumber, sliced
- 1 bell pepper, sliced
- 1 red onion, sliced
- 1 avocado, pitted, peeled and sliced
- 8 ounces goat cheese, crumbled

1. Heat the canola oil in a skillet over the highest heat. Once hot, carefully crack the eggs into the oil. Cook for 1 minute and flip the eggs using a wide spatula.
2. Fry the eggs until the yolks are set; reserve.
3. Mix the lettuce, cucumber, bell pepper, onion, and avocado in a serving bowl. Top with the fried eggs. Garnish with goat cheese and serve immediately. Bon appétit!

Per Serving

Calories: **474** | Fat: **38g** | Carbs: **6.3g** | Protein: **24g** | Fiber: **4.2g**

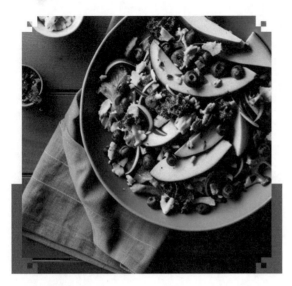
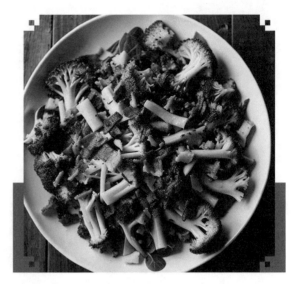

TURKEY-APPLE-WALNUT KALE SALAD

Prep time: 10 minutes | Cook time: 15 minutes | Serves 2

- 4 cups chopped kale
- ½ avocado, cubed
- ¼ red onion , finely chopped
- ¼ cup blueberries
- 2 tablespoons chopped and toasted walnuts
- ½ medium apple , cubed
- 8 ounces roasted turkey, sliced
- 6 tablespoons Greek Yogurt and Honey Dressing

1. In a medium bowl, combine the kale and avocado and massage the avocado into the kale with your hands. Add the onion, blueberries, walnuts, apple, and turkey, and toss well.
2. In each of 2 airtight storage containers or jars, place about 2 cups of salad. In 2 small airtight storage containers, place 3 tablespoons of Greek Yogurt and Honey Dressing. To serve, mix the salad and dressing.

Per Serving

Calories: 419 | Fat: 13g | Protein: 44g | Carbs: 46g | Fiber: 8g

CREAMY BROCCOLI-BACON SALAD

Prep time: 10 minutes | Cook time: 10 minutes | Serves 2

- 6 bacon slices
- ½ pound fresh broccoli, cut into small florets
- ¼ cup sliced almonds
- 1/3 cup mayonnaise
- 1 tablespoon honey mustard dressing

1. In a large skillet over medium-high heat, cook the bacon on both sides until crispy, about 8 minutes. Transfer the bacon to a paper towel–lined plate to drain and cool for 5 minutes. When cool, break the bacon into crumbles.
2. In a large bowl, combine the broccoli with the almonds and bacon.
3. In a small bowl, mix together the mayonnaise and honey mustard.
4. Add the dressing to the broccoli salad, and toss to thoroughly combine.
5. Chill the salad for 1 hour or more before serving.

Per Serving

Calories: 549 | Fat: 49g | Carbs: 16g | Fiber: 5g | Protein: 16g

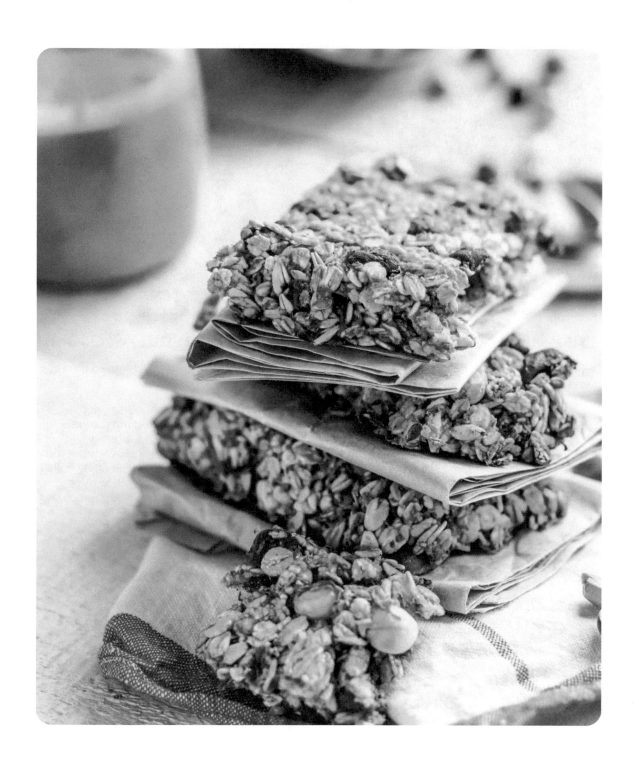

CHAPTER 9: SNACKS AND DESSERTS

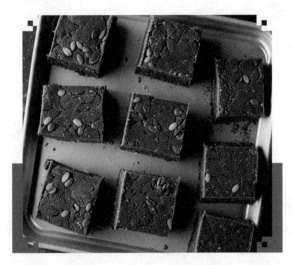
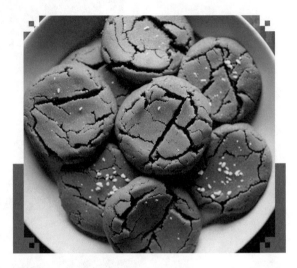

CAFÉ MOCHA PROTEIN BARS

Prep time: 5 minutes | **Cook time: 35 minutes** | **Serves 4**

- ¾ cup dry oatmeal
- ¼ cup oat bran
- 6 large egg whites
- 1 scoop chocolate protein powder
- ¼ teaspoon baking powder
- 1 teaspoon cocoa powder
- 1 tablespoon ground coffee
- 1 packet stevia

1. Preheat oven to 350°F.
2. Combine all ingredients in a blender and mix until smooth, then transfer to a greased 10" × 13" baking dish.
3. Bake 30 minutes and allow to cool before serving, cutting into 4 equal bars.

Per Serving

Calories: 127 | **Fat: 2 g** | **Protein: 15 g** | **Fiber: 3 g** | **Carbs: 15 g**

SALTED PEANUT BUTTER COOKIES

Prep time: 10 minutes | **Cook time: 40 minutes** | **Serves 4**

- 1 cup all-natural peanut butter (no added sugar)
- 1 cup granulated erythritol–monk fruit blend; less sweet: ½ cup
- 8 tablespoons (1 stick) unsalted butter, at room temperature
- 1 large egg, at room temperature
- 1 cup finely milled almond flour
- 1 teaspoon baking powder
- ½ teaspoon sea salt

1. Preheat the oven to 350°F. Line the baking sheet with parchment paper.
2. In the large bowl, using an electric mixer on medium high, combine the peanut butter, erythritol–monk fruit blend, butter, and egg and mix until combined, stopping and scraping the bowl once or twice, as needed. Add the almond flour and baking powder. Mix on low until fully incorporated.
3. Using a small cookie scoop or spoon, place tablespoon-size cookies on the prepared baking sheet and flatten them with the tines of a fork to make a crisscross design. Sprinkle the tops with the salt. Bake for 10 to 12 minutes, until lightly browned around the edges.
4. Allow the cookies to cool completely before eating.
5. Carefully handle these cookies when storing because they can be very fragile. They will last in the refrigerator for up to 5 days or in the freezer for up to 3 weeks.

Per Serving

Calories: 360 | **Fat: 32g** | **Carbs: 3g** | **Fiber: 2g** | **Protein: 11g**

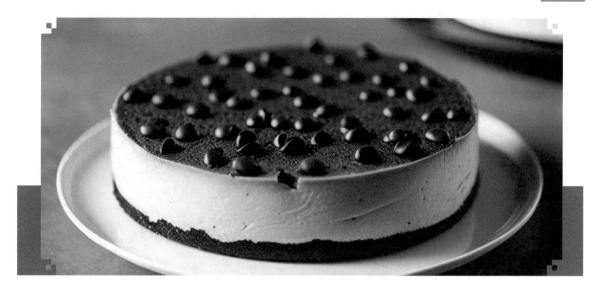

COOKIE FAT BOMBS

Prep time: 10 minutes | Cook time: 15 minutes | Serves 6

- 1 cup almond butter
- ½ cup coconut flour
- 1 teaspoon ground cinnamon
- ¼ cup cacao nibs or vegan keto chocolate chips

1. Line a baking sheet with parchment paper. If you don't have parchment paper, use aluminum foil or a greased pan.
2. In a mixing bowl, whisk together the almond butter, coconut flour, and cinnamon.
3. Fold in the cacao nibs.
4. Cover the bowl and put it in the freezer for 15 to 20 minutes.
5. Remove the bowl from the freezer and, using a spoon or cookie scoop, scoop out a dollop of mixture and roll it between your palms to form a ball. Repeat to use all the mixture.
6. Place the fat bombs on a baking sheet and put the sheet in the freezer to chill for 20 minutes until firm.

Per Serving

Calories: 319 | Fat: 26g | Carbs: 18g | Fiber: 10g | Protein: 8g

PROTEIN CHEESECAKE

Prep time: 5 minutes | Cook time: 10 minutes | Serves 12

- 24 ounces fat-free cream cheese
- ½ cup vanilla protein powder
- ¾ cup stevia
- 1 teaspoon vanilla extract
- 3 large eggs
- 1 tablespoon lemon juice
- 2 tablespoons semisweet chocolate chips

1. Preheat oven to 350°F. Spray a 9" pie pan with nonstick cooking spray.
2. Place cream cheese, protein powder, stevia, vanilla, eggs, and lemon juice in a large bowl and mix with a hand mixer on medium speed.
3. Pour mixture into the prepared pan. Sprinkle with chocolate chips.
4. Bake for 45 minutes. Remove from the oven and cool on a rack for 1 hour. Refrigerate for at least 3 hours before serving.

Per Serving

Calories: 126 | Fat: 4g | Carbs: 8g | Fiber: 8g | Protein: 14g

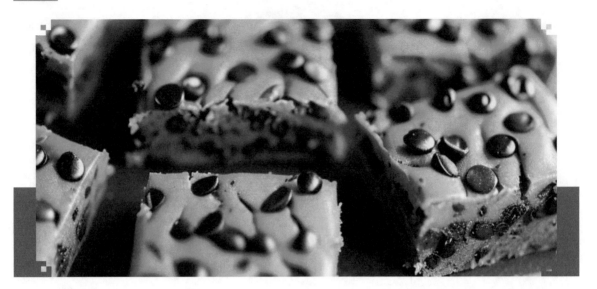

CHOCOLATE-AVOCADO PUDDING

Prep time: 5 minutes | Cook time: 10 minutes | Serves 3

- 1 ripe medium avocado, cut into chunks
- 2 ounces cream cheese, at room temperature
- 1 tablespoon Swerve natural sweetener
- 4 tablespoons unsweetened cocoa powder
- ¼ teaspoon vanilla extract
- Pinch pink Himalayan salt

1. In a food processor (or blender), combine the avocado with the cream cheese, sweetener, cocoa powder, vanilla, and pink Himalayan salt. Blend until completely smooth.
2. Pour into two small dessert bowls, and chill for 30 minutes before serving.

Per Serving

Calories: 281 | Fat: 27g | Carbs: 27g | Fiber: 10g | Protein: 8g

NO-BAKE PUMPKIN PROTEIN BARS

Prep time: 5 minutes | Cook time: 10 minutes | Serves 8

- ½ cup coconut flour
- ¼ cup vanilla protein powder
- ¾ teaspoon pumpkin pie spice
- ½ cup smooth almond butter
- ⅓ cup maple syrup
- 1 teaspoon vanilla extract
- ½ cup canned pumpkin purée
- 1 tablespoon unsweetened almond milk
- ½ cup semisweet chocolate chips

1. Line an 8" × 8" baking pan with parchment paper.
2. In a large bowl, combine coconut flour, protein powder, and pumpkin pie spice.
3. Place almond butter, maple syrup, and vanilla in a small saucepan. Heat over low heat, stirring constantly, until melted and combined, about 3 minutes.
4. Add almond butter mixture to the flour mixture and stir to combine. Add pumpkin and milk and stir until combined. Fold in chocolate chips. (The dough will be very thick.)
5. Transfer the dough to the prepared pan and press firmly with a spatula to pack the dough evenly across the pan. Refrigerate for at least 30 minutes.
6. Slice into eight bars and serve.

Per Serving

Calories: 246 | Fat: 12g | Carbs: 28g | Fiber: 6g | Protein: 7g

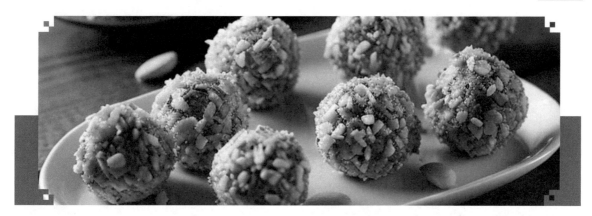

CHOCOLATE-DIPPED PEANUT BUTTER ICE POPS

Prep time: 10 minutes | Cook time: 5 minutes | Serves 12

- 8 ounces full-fat cream cheese, at room temperature
- 1 cup all-natural peanut butter (no added sugar or salt)
- ¼ cup confectioners' erythritol–monk fruit blend; less sweet: 2 tablespoons
- 1 teaspoon vanilla extract
- ¼ teaspoon sea salt
- 2 cups heavy (whipping) cream
- 4 ounces sugar-free chocolate chips
- 2 tablespoons coconut oil

1. In the large bowl, using an electric mixer on medium high, beat the cream cheese, peanut butter, confectioners' erythritol–monk fruit blend, vanilla, and salt. Add the heavy cream and combine until well incorporated.
2. Pour the mixture into the popsicle molds and add the popsicle sticks. Freeze for 3 to 4 hours, until frozen solid.
3. In the microwave-safe bowl, melt the chocolate baking chips and coconut oil in the microwave in 30-second intervals. Cool for 5 to 10 minutes.
4. Line the baking sheet with parchment paper. Dip the unmolded pops halfway into the melted chocolate, then place them on the prepared sheet and return them to the freezer for about 20 minutes. Store in the freezer in an airtight (nonglass) container for up to 3 weeks.

Per Serving

Calories: **405** | Fat: **37g** | Carbs: **9g** | Fiber: **3g** | Protein: **9g**

GOURMET "CHEESE" BALLS

Prep time: **1 hour 20 minutes** | Cook time: 15 minutes | Serves 6

- 1 cup raw hazelnuts, soaked overnight
- ¼ cup water
- 2 tablespoons nutritional yeast
- 1 teaspoon apple cider vinegar
- 1 teaspoon miso paste
- 1 teaspoon mustard
- ½ cup almond flour
- 1 cup slivered almonds
- 1 teaspoon dried oregano

1. In a high-powered blender, combine the hazelnuts, water, nutritional yeast, vinegar, miso paste, and mustard, and blend until well combined, thick, and creamy.
2. Transfer the mixture to a medium bowl.
3. Slowly stir in the almond flour until the mixture forms a dough-like consistency. Set aside.
4. In a separate, small bowl, toss the almonds and oregano together and set aside.
5. Using a soup spoon or tablespoon, scoop some mixture into your hand and shape it into a bite-size ball. Place the ball on a baking sheet. Repeat until you have used all the mixture (about 2 dozen balls).
6. One by one, roll the hazelnut balls in the almond and oregano mixture until thoroughly coated, placing each coated ball back on the baking sheet.
7. Place the sheet in the refrigerator for 1 hour to allow the balls to set.

Per Serving

Calories: **308** | Fat: **27g** | Carbs: **11g** | Fiber: **6g** | Protein: **10g**

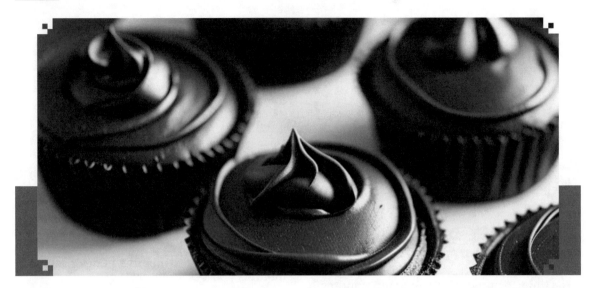

LEMON-POPPYSEED COOKIES

Prep time: 5 minutes | Cook time: 15 minutes | Serves 4

- Nonstick cooking spray
- 1 cup almond butter
- ¾ cup monk fruit sweetener
- 4 tablespoons chia seeds
- 3 tablespoons fresh grated lemon zest
- Juice of 1 lemon
- 1 tablespoon poppy seeds

1. Preheat the oven to 350°F. Grease a baking sheet with cooking spray and set aside.
2. In a large mixing bowl, combine the almond butter with the monk fruit sweetener, chia seeds, lemon zest, lemon juice, and poppy seeds. Mix well, kneading the mixture with your hands.
3. Roll pieces of the dough into cookie-size balls and place them on the prepared baking sheet, spacing them evenly, as some spreading will occur during baking
4. Bake the cookies for 8 minutes, until golden.
5. Transfer the cookies to a cooling rack.
6. Serve as is or paired with your favorite unsweetened, plant-based milk.

Per Serving

Calories: 460 | Fat: 39g | Carbs: 21g | Fiber: 12g | Protein: 13g

CHOCOLATE MOUSSE PIE CUPS

Prep time: 10 minutes | Cook time: 15 minutes | Serves 6

- ¾ cup coconut flour
- 2 flax "eggs"
- ½ cup coconut oil
- 4 avocados, peeled, pitted, and chopped
- 4 tablespoons cacao powder
- 3 tablespoons monk fruit sweetener
- Sea salt

1. Fill the cups of a muffin tin with cupcake liners.
2. In a large mixing bowl, combine the coconut flour, flax "eggs," and coconut oil. Mix thoroughly until you have a workable dough.
3. Scoop the dough a tablespoon at a time into the bottom of the cupcake liners, pressing it firmly to create a crust.
4. Place the muffin tin in the refrigerator for 1 hour to allow the crusts to firm up while you create the pie filling
5. In a large mixing bowl, combine the avocados, cacao powder, and monk fruit sweetener. Whip with a hand mixer on high until the mixture is well blended and airy.
6. Remove the muffin tin from refrigerator and divide the chocolate mousse mixture equally onto the prepared pie crusts.
7. Place the tin back in the refrigerator to set for 20 to 30 minutes before serving.

Per Serving

Calories: 439 | Fat: 39g | Carbs: 24g | Fiber: 16g | Protein: 6g

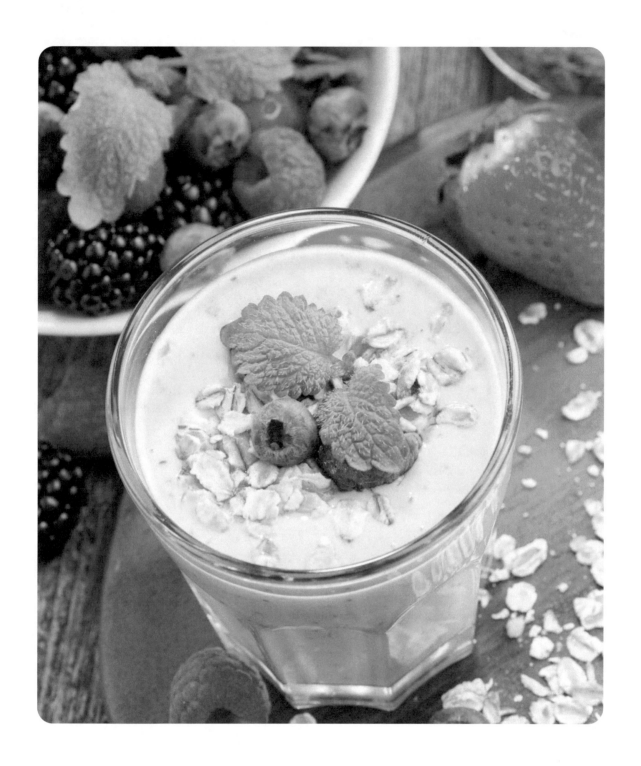

CHAPTER 10: HOMEMADE PROTEIN DRINKS

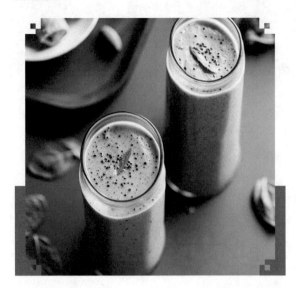

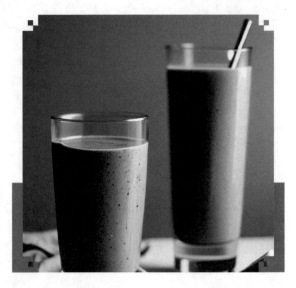

CREAMY COCONUT KIWI DRINK

Prep time: 3 minutes | Cook time: 3 minutes | Serves 4

- 5 kiwis, pulp scooped
- 2 tbsp erythritol
- 2 cups unsweetened coconut milk
- 2 cups coconut cream
- 7 ice cubes
- Mint leaves to garnish

1. In a blender, process the kiwis, erythritol, milk, cream, and ice cubes until smooth, about 3 minutes.
2. Pour into four serving glasses, garnish with mint leaves, and serve.

Per Serving

Calories: 351 | Fat: 28g | Carbs: 9.7g| Fiber: 3.5g | Protein: 16g

BERRY GREEN SMOOTHIE

Prep time: 10 minutes | Cook time: 15 minutes | Serves 2

- 1 cup water
- ½ cup raspberries
- ½ cup shredded kale
- ¾ cup cream cheese
- 1 tablespoon coconut oil
- 1 scoop vanilla protein powder

1. Put the water, raspberries, kale, cream cheese, coconut oil, and protein powder in a blender and blend until smooth.
2. Pour into 2 glasses and serve immediately.

Per Serving

Calories: 436 | Fat: 36g | Protein: 28g | Carbs: 11g | Fiber: 5g

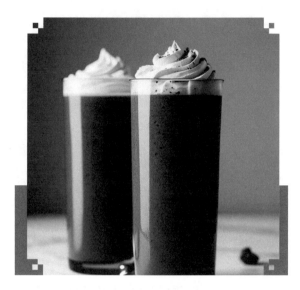

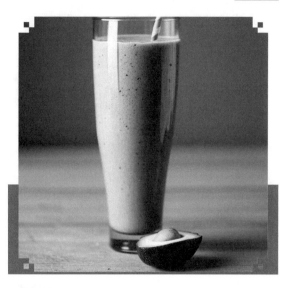

COFFEE SMOOTHIE

Prep time: 5 minutes | Cook time: 15 minutes | Serves 2

- 1 cup unsweetened hemp milk
- ½ cup ice
- 1/3 cup cold-brew coffee
- ½ avocado
- 2 tablespoons cacao powder
- 1 scoop plant-based, low-carb protein powder (such as Truvani or Sunwarrior brands) (optional)
- 2 or 3 drops liquid stevia

1. Combine all the ingredients in a blender and blend on high until creamy and smooth.
2. Divide between tall serving glasses and enjoy chilled.

Per Serving

Calories: **130** | Fat: **9g** | Carbs: **8g** | Fiber: **4g** |Protein: **3g**

GREEN COLLAGEN SMOOTHIE

Prep time: 5 minutes | Cook time: 10 minutes | Serves 1

- 2 cups baby spinach
- ½ medium avocado, peeled and pitted
- ½ medium banana, peeled and frozen
- ¼ cup collagen powder
- 1 cup unsweetened almond milk

1. Combine all ingredients in a blender and process until smooth.
2. Pour into a tall glass and serve immediately.

Per Serving

Calories: **356** | Fat: **13g** | Carbs: **25g** | Fiber: **9g** | Protein: **37g**

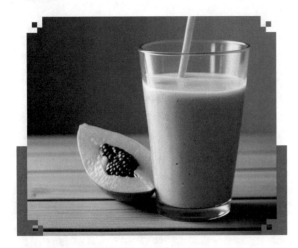

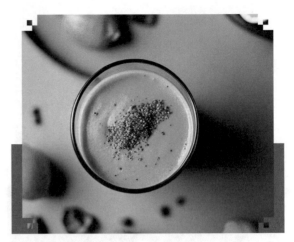

SUNNY CITRUS SMOOTHIE

Prep time: 5 minutes | Cook time: 15 minutes | Serves 5

For The Smoothie Packs:

- 1¼ cups frozen pineapple chunks, divided
- 1¼ cups frozen papaya chunks, divided
- 1¼ cups frozen mango chunks, divided
- 2½ fresh or frozen bananas, chopped (300g), divided
- 2½ tablespoons ground flaxseed, divided

For The Smoothies:

- 2½ cups nonfat vanilla greek yogurt, divided
- 2½ cups orange juice, divided

To Make The Smoothie Packs:

1. Into each of 5 resealable freezer bags, place ¼ cup of pineapple, ¼ cup of papaya, ¼ cup of mango, half a banana, and ½ tablespoon of flaxseed. Flatten, pressing any air out of the bag, and seal. Store in the freezer until ready to use.

To Make A Smoothie:

1. In a blender, combine ½ cup of yogurt, ½ cup of orange juice, and the contents of 1 smoothie pack, and blend until smooth.

Per Serving

Calories: 273 | Fat: 2g | Protein: 13g | Carbs: 63g | Fiber: 5g

ORANGE JULIUS SMOOTHIE

Prep time: 5 minutes | Cook time: 15 minutes | Serves 2

For The Smoothie Packs:

- 1 cup (90g) frozen mango chunks, divided
- 1 cup (50g) chopped baby carrots, divided
- 1 fresh or frozen banana (118g), chopped, divided
- 1 scoop (30g) vanilla vegan protein powder, divided
- 2 tablespoons (10g) hemp hearts, divided
- 8 to 12 ice cubes, divided

For The Smoothies:

- ½ cup (120ml) orange juice, divided
- ½ cup (120ml) unsweetened almond milk, divided

To Make The Smoothie Packs:

1. In each of 2 resealable freezer bags, combine ½ cup of mango, ¼ cup of carrots, half a banana, ½ scoop of protein powder, 1 tablespoon of hemp hearts, and 4 to 6 ice cubes. Lay the bags flat and remove as much air as possible before sealing. Store in the freezer until ready to use.

To Make A Smoothie:

1. In a blender, combine 1 smoothie pack with ¼ cup of orange juice and ¼ cup of almond milk. Blend well.

Per Serving

Calories: 352 | Fat: 15g | Protein: 21g | Carbs: 44g | Fiber: 7g

APPENDIX 1: MEASUREMENT CONVERSION CHART

MEASUREMENT CONVERSION CHART

VOLUME EQUIVALENTS(DRY)

US STANDARD	METRIC (APPROXIMATE)
1/8 teaspoon	0.5 mL
1/4 teaspoon	1 mL
1/2 teaspoon	2 mL
3/4 teaspoon	4 mL
1 teaspoon	5 mL
1 tablespoon	15 mL
1/4 cup	59 mL
1/2 cup	118 mL
3/4 cup	177 mL
1 cup	235 mL
2 cups	475 mL
3 cups	700 mL
4 cups	1 L

WEIGHT EQUIVALENTS

US STANDARD	METRIC (APPROXIMATE)
1 ounce	28 g
2 ounces	57 g
5 ounces	142 g
10 ounces	284 g
15 ounces	425 g
16 ounces (1 pound)	455 g
1.5 pounds	680 g
2 pounds	907 g

VOLUME EQUIVALENTS(LIQUID)

US STANDARD	US STANDARD (OUNCES)	METRIC (APPROXIMATE)
2 tablespoons	1 fl.oz.	30 mL
1/4 cup	2 fl.oz.	60 mL
1/2 cup	4 fl.oz.	120 mL
1 cup	8 fl.oz.	240 mL
1 1/2 cup	12 fl.oz.	355 mL
2 cups or 1 pint	16 fl.oz.	475 mL
4 cups or 1 quart	32 fl.oz.	1 L
1 gallon	128 fl.oz.	4 L

TEMPERATURES EQUIVALENTS

FAHRENHEIT(F)	CELSIUS(C) (APPROXIMATE)
225 °F	107 °C
250 °F	120 °C
275 °F	135 °C
300 °F	150 °C
325 °F	160 °C
350 °F	180 °C
375 °F	190 °C
400 °F	205 °C
425 °F	220 °C
450 °F	235 °C
475 °F	245 °C
500 °F	260 °C

The Dirty Dozen and Clean Fifteen

The Environmental Working Group (EWG) is a nonprofit, nonpartisan organization dedicated to protecting human health and the environment Its mission is to empower people to live healthier lives in a healthier environment. This organization publishes an annual list of the twelve kinds of produce, in sequence, that have the highest amount of pesticide residue-the Dirty Dozen-as well as a list of the fifteen kinds ofproduce that have the least amount of pesticide residue-the Clean Fifteen.

THE DIRTY DOZEN

- The 2016 Dirty Dozen includes the following produce. These are considered among the year's most important produce to buy organic:

Strawberries	Spinach
Apples	Tomatoes
Nectarines	Bell peppers
Peaches	Cherry tomatoes
Celery	Cucumbers
Grapes	Kale/collard greens
Cherries	Hot peppers

- *The Dirty Dozen list contains two additional itemskale/collard greens and hot peppers-because they tend to contain trace levels of highly hazardous pesticides.*

THE CLEAN FIFTEEN

- The least critical to buy organically are the Clean Fifteen list. The following are on the 2016 list:

Avocados	Papayas
Corn	Kiw
Pineapples	Eggplant
Cabbage	Honeydew
Sweet peas	Grapefruit
Onions	Cantaloupe
Asparagus	Cauliflower
Mangos	

- *Some of the sweet corn sold in the United States are made from genetically engineered (GE) seedstock. Buy organic varieties of these crops to avoid GE produce.*

APPENDIX 3: INDEX

Hey there!

Wow, can you believe we've reached the end of this culinary journey together? I'm truly thrilled and filled with joy as I think back on all the recipes we've shared and the flavors we've discovered. This experience, blending a bit of tradition with our own unique twists, has been a journey of love for good food. And knowing you've been out there, giving these dishes a try, has made this adventure incredibly special to me.

Even though we're turning the last page of this book, I hope our conversation about all things delicious doesn't have to end. I cherish your thoughts, your experiments, and yes, even those moments when things didn't go as planned. Every piece of feedback you share is invaluable, helping to enrich this experience for us all.

I'd be so grateful if you could take a moment to share your thoughts with me, be it through a review on Amazon or any other place you feel comfortable expressing yourself online. Whether it's praise, constructive criticism, or even an idea for how we might do things differently in the future, your input is what truly makes this journey meaningful.

This book is a piece of my heart, offered to you with all the love and enthusiasm I have for cooking. But it's your engagement and your words that elevate it to something truly extraordinary.

Thank you from the bottom of my heart for being such an integral part of this culinary adventure. Your openness to trying new things and sharing your experiences has been the greatest gift.

Catch you later,

Betty J. Lawson

Made in United States
Troutdale, OR
12/08/2024